The Compassionate Caregiver's Guide to Caring for Someone with Cancer

by

Bonnie Bajorek Daneker

Bloomington, IN Milton Keynes, UK

authorHOUSE®

AuthorHouse™
1663 Liberty Drive, Suite 200
Bloomington, IN 47403
www.authorhouse.com
Phone: 1-800-839-8640

AuthorHouse™ UK Ltd.
500 Avebury Boulevard
Central Milton Keynes, MK9 2BE
www.authorhouse.co.uk
Phone: 08001974150

First published by AuthorHouse 4/2/2007

ISBN: 978-1-4259-8974-3 (sc)

Library of Congress Control Number: 2007902131

Printed in the United States of America
Bloomington, Indiana

This book is printed on acid-free paper.

For those impacted by cancer worldwide,

especially my fellow caregivers

Table of Contents

Acknowledgments

I am deeply grateful to the dozens of patients and caregivers who shared their stories with me. Their tales of challenge and joy showed me that I was not alone. Their love and selflessness continue to inspire me.

Since I began work on this book years ago, many accomplished professionals have guided me on content. These amazing people comprise The Compassionate Caregiver's Medical Advisory Board. They have willingly given me their precious time, knowledge and encouragement, and I cannot thank them enough. Their input will appear in this book, in the upcoming workbooks and handbooks, and throughout my web site. They are:

Andrew Toledo, MD; Angel Blanco, MD; Annette Brooks-Warren, MD; Beth Horwicz, RN; Bonnie Tillman, RN, BSN; Brad Pohlman, MD; Brenda Fulp, RN, LCP, EdS, NCC; C. Daniel Allen, MD; Caroline Horne, DMV, PA-C; Cheryl Hiddleson, RN; Deb Eikey, RN, OCN, CHPN; Gary Bernstein, MD; George Daneker, MD, FACS; George Warsaw, PhD; Jennifer Buckley, RN; Jerry Porter, MD; John Davis, PhD; John Robinson, MD; Kay Payne, CST; Laura Williams, RN; Linda Stamm, PhD; Melissa Hall, PA-C, RD; Melissa LeBouef, BSN; Meredith Shelley, RN, OCN; Metta Johnson, RN, BSN, OCN, CHPN; R.C. Brownlow, MD; Rachel Boersma, PhD(c), BSN, RN, MS, CARN; Renee Sevy Rickles, LMSW; Ron Steis, MD; Sandra Parker, RN, CNP; and Steve Curley, MD, FACS. Special commendation goes to Gary Bernstein, Jennifer Buckley and Melissa LeBoeuf. They persisted with me through multiple interviews and drafts. I think they are angels in earthly form.

The staffs at the Cleveland Clinic (Cleveland, Ohio location), Taussig Cancer Center, Akron General Medical Center, Akron City Hospital, and Wadsworth-Rittman Hospital have earned a special place in my heart for their skilled, direct, compassionate care of my father. The lovely greeters at the Taussig Cancer Center always had a wheelchair and a smile at the ready. Mike Bianco, MD deserves an award for sticking with my family, even through the "Impossible Patient" days.

The Cancer Survivor's Network at Saint Joseph's Hospital in Atlanta was my first formal support group and it now provides a wonderful way to serve this community. I am honored.

Melissa Rosati patiently coached me through the writing and publishing process. Suzanne Adair Williams published her book ahead of me, becoming a beacon in the quagmire. Kathleen Kiley offered a spot on her television show. As a friend, she also offered peace of mind and accountability as we worked on our manuscripts at the same time.

My editor and friend, Julie Simon, understands the meaning of "catharsis." God bless her. With her, I brainstormed ideas, questioned the outline, and reworked much of the book. It wouldn't be in its present form without her.

My clients and employers provided flexibility and understanding to bring this idea to life, for which I am indebted.

Many other friends have offered help in a variety of capacities: editing, advising, marketing, researching, and listening. Thank you.

Speaking of listening, I must mention my brothers and sisters. They've heard me talk about this book for years and now it's finally here. Though some were more involved than others on this project, all were full of advice and encouragement. Chris was my "sidekick" on this caregiving journey; whether I needed a kick in the pants or a friend at my side, she was there, another angel in my midst. "Thank you" doesn't even come close to cutting it.

I used to say I got my strength from my dad and my spice from my mom. Now I see I got strength from my mom as well. She understood what I was feeling and never failed to encourage me to finish this book. Keep going strong, Mom! I know my father continues to be with us in spirit and I want both of you around.

I'd like to thank Spencer, Elliot, and Matthew for offering the support they could, never having met my father.

Saving the best for last: my precious treasure. My husband helped create the loving, healing environment I needed at times of great loss. The combination of his personal and professional interests in this book added dimensions I could not have included alone. Many late nights were spent editing each page of this manuscript, which we affectionately call "The Encyclopedia of Caregiving" and I will forever remember that. I couldn't ask for a better partner to share my vision and my life. Thank you.

Introduction

The call came on that October evening at 6:42 p.m.

I remember the time exactly, as many of us do, when we hear about a cancer diagnosis.

"It doesn't look good, Bon," said my brother. This immediately put me on alert. A doctor himself, he usually tempered bad news. His next comment— "They've given him eight weeks to live"—sent me into panic. I looked at the clock, as if I could stop time by staring at the numbers. 6,4,2.

The activities of my normally fast-paced life suddenly seemed unimportant. I had been out of town and was eager to make up lost time in my professional and social life upon my return. But that eagerness left me. I asked my brother for more details. Though we'd been unaware of it, my father had been experiencing night sweats for months. It wasn't worrisome during the hot summer. When they increased in frequency and severity through September, he and my mother knew something was wrong.

They went to the doctor for tests, which identified it as Non-Hodgkin's Lymphoma, Aggressive Diffuse Large B-Cell Lymphoma, my brother said.

There must be some mistake, I was thinking. My dad's never sick. It's probably been forty years since he was in the hospital. Reading my thoughts, my brother said it looked like he would be spending some time there now and I may want to go up and see him.

Of course I would. It was just a question of when. With my job and other responsibilities I had some flexibility, a luxury most of my family did not have. In a few days, I was on an airplane to begin my caregiving experience. The trip across four states was one with which I was going to become very familiar.

My caregiving experience did not last eight weeks. I prefer to think that the disease did not know what a rival it would have in my father. He fought different types of cancer, one after another. He endured test after test. He had treatment after treatment. He was determined to be as aggressive about staying alive as the cancer was about claiming him. He was with us for four more years.

I am thankful and humbled to have been a primary caregiver. Thankful to return care to someone who had cared for me growing up. Humbled to watch a pillar in my life struggle to survive. Though I could do many things, I could not take his cancer away.

Cancer is a hugely powerful disease with far-reaching impacts. It can alter relationships, overturn finances and destroy careers. It can steal rational thinking and sap physical strength in caregivers and patients alike. It can push friends and family into emotional turmoil and heated decision-making. I have witnessed all of this.

During those years, my own life seemed fragmented as I existed in two cities. While I was doing my best to stay connected in both places, I never felt fully "present" in either. When in one place, I was aware of my responsibilities at the other and vice versa. There was always something that needed to be done. I needed help.

I read books, articles, and web sites to help me understand the diseases. I found nothing that told me what to expect, how I could plan for it, and how I could involve others for the patient's benefit. I certainly found no encouragement to take care of myself.

Talking to other caregivers in the waiting rooms, I realized they needed the same type of help. They had the same challenges with lifestyle changes, relationships, job responsibilities, and spirituality. We commiserated. We compared solutions to home problems with eating, moving, dressing, and washing.

I said earlier that I could not take my father's cancer away. Listening to fellow caregivers showed me that I *could* counter some of the negative impacts of this disease. I *could* help other caregivers on their journey by sharing what we had all learned the hard way. Those informal conversations became a collection of recommendations and so The Compassionate Caregiver Series® began.

After the second year of his illness, I started to outline my approach and to begin formal interviews. I involved medical professionals who were familiar with my father's case, as well as others from various connections. They became the Medical Advisory Board for the series. They universally supported my efforts and guided me on filling the medical gaps.

The Compassionate Caregiver's Guide to Caring for Someone with Cancer itself is a work of compassion. I have written this book to prepare you for your journey and to help you to be an effective caregiver. I have written it for the cancer patients too, in hopes that they will benefit from your compassionate, effective care.

I've included tools to help with a variety of situations. You'll find planning checklists, phrases to communicate with medical professionals, and strategies to care for yourself. You'll also see recommendations from fellow caregivers throughout the book.

It will help if you're aware of a few conventions:

- I have written this book for the adult cancer patient and caregiver. Some subject matter related to intimacy, fertility, and sexuality may not be as appropriate for younger readers.

- I believe that childhood cancers and challenges with growing up are worthy of their own book title. This is likely to become part of The Compassionate Caregiver Series® at a later date.

- I have generally decided to use "patient" throughout the book to avoid potentially incorrect phrasing such as "spouse," "loved one," or "friend."

- The medical professionals who are usually involved in administering the traditional treatments are described in Chapter 3. Other professionals who may be consulted are described as well. For the purpose of consistency, I have used male pronouns to describe the doctors.

- Because cancer does not discriminate, I've included examples from patients and caregivers in many demographics. The text following those examples contains pronouns that reflect the gender of the person in the example.

- To protect the privacy of some interviewees, I have honored their requests and changed or omitted names in some quotes or comments. While most are verbatim from individual caregivers, some are composites from multiple people.

- In the time it took to complete and publish this book, many gifted researchers have made discoveries and advances in oncology and cancer care. I hope to include them as updates in future versions of this book.

With that in mind, please remember that this book is not intended as a substitute for medical advice or to endorse a specific course of action related to treatment. That advice should be obtained from the doctor who is familiar with and responsible for the patient's care. If you have a question about the recommendations in this book in relation to the patient, be sure to check with the doctor.

This book refers to cancer as a single diagnosis. In reality, a cancer diagnosis is often compounded by other serious considerations, including:

- Financial impact, such as the loss of a primary breadwinner and benefits provider

- Familial impact, when the patient is a child or when children lose a parent/guardian

- Emotional challenges, when there is a death closely following another loss such as a death, divorce, or diagnosis of another illness

- Physical and mental challenges.

If these fit your situation, you should actively look for support from professionals who are specifically trained in these areas, support groups, or books on the subject.

Finally, this book is a partnership. Please send your suggestions and ideas for continuous improvement. Visit the web site at www.CompassionateCaregiverOnline.com or send an email to me at bonnie@CompassionateCaregiverOnline.com. Let me know what other tools or support you need on your caregiving journey.

In health,

Bonnie Bajorek Daneker
Fellow Caregiver

Chapter 1: Becoming a Caregiver

"I'm not sure I'm the right person for the job," says Doug, 70. "My wife has always looked after me. But now she has breast cancer and needs me to care for her. It's hard to admit that I have no idea what to do or even who to talk to about such a sensitive subject. Where do I start?"

First, congratulations to you for picking up this book. You've recognized that someone you care about is having a health problem and you want to help. Without realizing it, you've taken the first step toward becoming a compassionate, effective caregiver.

No matter what your relationship to the patient is, you can help. No matter how extensive your prior experience with the medical condition is, you can help. However, you will need reliable information about the different forms that caregiving may take and you will need to make decisions about how you want to help.

Many serious diseases strike without warning. The opportunity to be a caregiver usually comes about unexpectedly and when it does, friends and family members commonly react in one of three ways:

1. Some immediately take on the role, without necessarily knowing what it entails.

2. Others recognize that they do not know what the responsibilities are and they investigate what needs to be done to best help the patient.

3. Still others dismiss the idea, having no interest or doubting their own abilities.

The Compassionate Caregiver's Guide to Caring for Someone with Cancer is designed for those who are willing to be involved in the cancer patient's care on any level. This book will enable you to grasp your new position as caregiver and to manage the lifestyle impacts that sometimes accompany caregiving. It will also show you ways to provide good care to a cancer patient while maintaining your own health.

The goal of this chapter is to give an overview of the caregiver responsibilities that you may face. We'll help you:

- Understand What It Means to Be a Caregiver to a Cancer Patient

- Identify the Roles You May Play as a Caregiver

- Recognize Common Impacts to Major Areas of Your Life

- Set Up for Success

- Take Care of Yourself.

Throughout this book, we'll be making choices and setting expectations for the caregiving process. Sections entitled "What Do I Say?" and "How Can I Help?" appear along the way to give you guidance, as well as helpful quotes from fellow caregivers. When the patient's need for you lessens, we'll look at post-treatment survivorship. Then, we'll form new goals for healthy living as the book comes to a close.

So, let's get started.

Understanding What It Means to be a Caregiver to a Cancer Patient

"They called me his 'caregiver' at the hospital," says Beth, 55. "I've never been called that before. I guess that's what I am. I mean, I'm not his spouse or daughter, just a neighbor. But when I heard he had lung cancer, I went to help out. He's been so good to us. He needed somebody and I don't know where the rest of his family is, so here I am."

Devoting your time and attention to someone with cancer is an incredible gift to them. Caregiving for patients with serious illnesses maintains their comfort and their ability to function. It adds to their emotional and physical well-being and it enhances the quality of their life.

Being a caregiver means that you must continually evaluate what the patient can and cannot do – and help when help is needed. You'll need to sometimes be the patient's advocate and conscience to make the most of medical advice.

Caregiving is not a responsibility to be taken lightly. Cancer patients are sick with a serious illness and you may see painful deterioration of their physical or mental capabilities from the disease or treatments. You may see their personality and your relationship diminished. You must be ready to assist in a variety of circumstances that are not glamorous and are often taxing. It can be a delicate balance between lending a hand where needed and not stepping in to straighten out the patient's life.

Additional challenges, like the uncertainty of how long the "assignment" is and the possibility of complications, may arise. When you take on caregiving responsibilities – regardless of how involved they are – you will not know when the patient will return to independent living. Nor will you be able to predict how other illnesses, a history of past harmful behaviors, or other physical considerations can complicate how this illness will be managed. This is not to say that you will be taking on all of this yourself.

Patients can, and often do, have multiple caregivers. In addition to medically-trained personnel at care facilities, one person becomes the main contact. This person, usually a spouse/partner or family member, becomes the "primary" caregiver. Other caregivers fulfill responsibilities as the patient's needs change, often supporting the primary caregiver. The following pages take a look at these responsibilities and outline various roles you may play as a caregiver.

Identifying Roles You May Play as a Caregiver

"In some ways, it's like being a parent," says Paulette, 37, who cares for her grandmother with colon cancer. "I'm her gopher, driver, cook, and housekeeper. I help her to eat and encourage her. I take care of her pets and her finances. I know she just can't do very much without me."

When you hear that a friend or relative is having a health problem, you may wonder what you will be called on to do as a caregiver. Chances are, you haven't had this experience before and you don't know what it entails. While each patient and each disease is different, there are generalities that you will likely face. Knowing what may be expected of you will help to prepare you for taking on those roles and responsibilities.

In the quote above, Paulette talks about some of the more obvious roles in caregiving. Others may not be so obvious. Take a look at the descriptions below that have been provided by other caregivers of cancer patients. When you read these descriptions, try to envision yourself in the roles.

- ***Primary Caregiver*** – A primary caregiver addresses the majority of the patient's needs at home or in transit and you may be taking on many of the patient's medical and non-medical needs. You will probably be the center of the support network and become the point of contact for communications. Because of this, you may find yourself delegating responsibilities and supervising others.

  Every primary caregiver needs a back-up, though. This back-up can take over the responsibilities for a time and give the primary caregiver some rest. While you may not need a back-up often, it's vital to prevent burnout and depression. This replacement can be someone local or out of town, as long as she can travel in when you need her.

- ***Interface to Medical Professionals*** – Getting to know the patient's healthcare providers is crucial to understanding her care. As an interface, you may find yourself:

  o Writing down appointment times and attending those appointments

  o Leading interactions with medical professionals, taking notes to review later, learning a new "vocabulary," and speaking on behalf of the patient

  o Acting as an informed advisor to the patient and keeping track of the patient's medical information.

- ***Information Gatherer*** –You'll both be learning faster than cramming for an important test. As a student learning about the illness and as an educator teaching others, you'll likely come across a variety of resources: books, the internet, journal articles, conferences, and support groups. Be wary of the reliability of the information before you act on it.

- *Record Keeper* – Some people are detailed-oriented and some are not. With the amount of paper that accompanies an insurance claim, you need to identify someone to coordinate administrative issues.

- *Spokesperson* – As a weekly/daily reporter, you may become a strategic messenger who delivers updates on the situation. It will be a challenge to decide what details and contact information to share with family members and well wishers. In this role, you may monitor visitors as well.

- *Medication Manager* – You may need to encourage/remind the patient to take medicines. Trying to remember which medicines to give, when to give them, and how to give them can keep you on your toes. You may need to assign someone to pick-up prescriptions and refills, as well as non-prescription items like lotions or ointments.

- *Mobility Expert* – If the patient is having difficulty moving, you may be called on to help her dress, go to the restroom, wash herself, get into the car, or walk a corridor. You may also be challenged with home adjustments or special equipment.

- *Legal Advisor* – Legal matters may surface in the form of patient rights, medical bill arbitration, end-of-life decision-making, and Healthcare Power of Attorney. Chapter 2 explains these issues.

After reading about these roles, you'll notice that some fit more comfortably than others. Mentally earmark the roles you'll more readily take on and earmark the others as potential for delegation. Realistically evaluate your ability to provide what is needed, especially if the caregiving needs are permanent or extensive. You do not have to take on all the roles yourself. You may want to enlist the help of a friend or professional caregiver. Don't be afraid to ask. That's why they are there.

The level of involvement in caregiving is a personal choice. If you cannot take on the role of the primary caregiver but would like to contribute, you can still help the patient. Offer to bring over a hot meal, run some errors, or watch the kids.

Whatever roles you decide to play, you'll want to sidestep some of the tolls they could take. The next sections focus on the possible impacts to your lifestyle. They are designed to help you maintain your own healthy outlook and stance as you care for the patient.

A Few Words on Repeating the Caregiving Experience

Those of you who have already had an especially difficult caregiving experience may not be eager to repeat it. However, you may want to think about this: the second time around may be easier than the first. If you've encountered similar situations before, you've probably found shortcuts and ways to multi-task or delegate what needs to be done. Because you know how to avoid the pitfalls, you can concentrate on making caregiving a very positive, loving experience.

Exploring Common Lifestyle Impacts

"Nobody tells you the bad parts of caregiving," says Molly, 35. "It's like having a baby – they don't focus on talking about the screaming through the night or dirty diapers. They just tell you instead about how nice of an experience it is and that they were happy they could do it."

When you are thinking about tending to someone with a health difficulty, understand that you'll become familiar with that difficulty. You will learn about the disease and probably meet others with similar challenges. As you take on the various caregiving roles and the patient's condition changes, you will experience impacts to major parts of your life.

If you recognize these common lifestyle impacts, you may be able to take precautions to minimize their effect on you. We'll look at possible areas of impact including:

- Family relationships

- Home and lifestyle

- Intimate relationships

- Work responsibilities

- Spirituality.

Striving to overcome any serious disease is a commitment because it affects both the caregiver and the patient. In later chapters, we'll address specific scenarios in which the disease and the treatment impact the patient but the next few sections are all about you, the caregiver.

Family Relationships

If you are related to the patient (by blood or by marriage), you will likely experience some change to the family dynamic, as these caregivers did:

> ➤ "The hardest part for me was the 'role reversal,' where I'm the son, but now I'm in charge, caring for my mom," says Tony, 39. "I've heard of this happening to non-medical persons taking care of sick nurses or doctors, too."

> ➤ "I found it extremely difficult to care for my grandfather and my sick child at the same time," says Lisa, 44. "They call it 'being part of the sandwich generation,' where you're caught in the middle of two people that need you. You cannot give 100% to everybody. They may feel slighted or left out when you're giving attention to the other one and there's virtually no time left for your own needs."

> "What I couldn't understand was the reaction of my siblings and other relatives," says Bryan, 52. "It was like they expected me to do everything. They were just not involved, unaware or uncaring. It didn't seem like they respected what I was doing. I certainly never heard the words 'thank you' from either them or our dad."

While it's true that caregiving may be challenging and that you may not be thanked for the wide range of activities you do on behalf of the patient, much good can come out of this experience for you on a personal level:

- You can become closer to the patient and potentially to other family members, as the priorities become family, health, and goodwill towards each other.

- You're given a chance to strengthen damaged relationships or bring closure to unresolved issues.

- You can encounter ways to show love where you may have been unable or unwilling to do so in the past.

Home and Lifestyle

If you are living in the same place as the patient, your personal space and routine may be compromised. That will require some adjustment and flexibility, like these caregivers found:

> "Ever since my sister was diagnosed and moved in, I cannot escape it," says Carrie, 52. "This illness interferes with my regular activities, and our relationship has not been the same. While I want to be helpful, I'm resentful. I want to get this unwanted stranger out – not my sister, but the cancer!"

> ➢ "I guess I shouldn't complain about his bed on first floor now or how the bathroom's been converted," says Henry, 60. "I've heard about people remodeling their whole house, with kitchen counters adjusted to the right heights and ramps or lifts for wheelchairs."

> ➢ "I've learned to eat what he eats, when he can eat," says Monica, 38. "It's so hard to guess what he'll be hungry for and when."

You may see your own situation above. But take heart, you may see some benefits:

- You'll likely become aware of your own nutrition and habits and you may make some positive changes.

- You'll be close enough to profit from advice of doctors and other specialists for use in your own health.

- If home adjustments are made, there may be an opportunity to incorporate changes that you would otherwise want.

Intimate Relationships

When a romantic partnership is involved, it's important to remember each other's vulnerability during this time and not exploit it. These caregivers relate their challenges about intimacy, sexuality and fertility with a partner with cancer:

> ➢ "Caregiving brings good and bad up to the forefront," says Edward, 70. "My wife and I are spending a lot of time together. The potential to open old emotional wounds or dust off skeletons from many years of marriage is definitely there."

> ➢ "I never dreamed that I would be weak and sore," says Joan, 59. "My husband's the one with cancer but moving, bathing, and dressing him are no small tasks. On top of everything else, they are straining our marriage. I'm going to get some assistance."

> ➢ "There are a lot of physical changes in my partner like weight loss, hair loss, general discoloration," says Kevin, 40. "Add to that nausea and vomiting and my libido pulls a disappearing act. We've got to do something."

> ➢ "I know we have to make decisions on treatment that may affect us having children or not," says Shelley, 30. "Do we have to do it this second? I can't think about that now."

While there may be awkwardness in communication, don't be ashamed to bring up how you feel about your private relationship to your partner. Think of the possible benefits:

- You've been given opportunities to be closer and more creative in your expressions of love. Think about how you can work around the obstacles.

- In trying new ways to communicate, you may have a chance to rediscover the person you fell in love with and learn to find solace in each other.

- You may pursue talking to a therapist about issues, both cancer-related and not.

Work Responsibilities

In addition to caring for someone with cancer, many caregivers continue to work at another job. Issues that surface affect workers at every level, from management to administrators. Managing two sets of responsibilities requires a great deal of balance and planning, as shown in these caregiver quotes:

> "I'm temporarily giving up career advancement for flexibility and less stress," says Andrew, 37. "After this caregiving gig is over, how can I get my career back on track?"

> "All of a sudden, I was the breadwinner," says Mina, 55. "I hadn't worked since being a teacher in our twenties. We had no other income but plenty of medical expenses. I was at a loss because I didn't know how to handle money matters. But I learned."

> "I'm afraid to talk about my home situation at work," says Anja, 34. "But I will need some explanation soon as to why I need to keep leaving for doctors' appointments, or why I'm having difficulty concentrating."

Many are reluctant to involve their work situation in their private matters, especially when it comes to an illness that often requires a lot of attention. If you do open up, though, you may be surprised to find:

- People's generosity at work can be helpful and even inspiring.

- A community of support may unveil solutions that would not otherwise be obvious to you.

- You have the opportunity to review your work position. While thinking about career options, you may discover a new vocation.

Spirituality

Spirituality is often a very private matter. Some people openly turn toward faith as a foundation of their life, while others may celebrate in limited ways or not at all. You may become more religious or less religious as a result of your caregiving experience as these caregivers report:

> ➤ "My faith is what got me through," says Carol, 55. "This experience just confirms what I already knew, that there is a greater power than me in control and everything happens for a reason."

> ➤ "I'm not sure why God did this to us. We're good people," says Les, 60. "It seems like all our prayers were good for nothing."

> ➤ "I never was much of a churchgoer but being around the chaplain at this hospital has made me interested again," says Gerald, 77.

Whatever your spiritual inclination, you may have an opportunity to support the patient's inclination as well. You may want to make this your spiritual goal: to build on your beliefs and continue confidently in a direction that is mentally, emotionally, and physically healthy for both you and the patient.

After you've taken a look at these common impacts to your spirituality, job situation, home life, and relationships, you'll have a better sense of what may happen in your caregiving journey. When you know about these in advance, you will be able to position yourself to avoid the negative and highlight the positive.

Making the Decision to be a Caregiver

"My best friend was diagnosed with breast cancer," says Dana, 39. "I kept thinking 'How do I help her without being condescending?' I want to let her know that I can do this because I care, not because I'm feeling sorry for her."

Given the possible lifestyle impacts and additional responsibilities, you may wonder why anyone would become a caregiver. Caregivers answer this question by saying that they thought they were the natural choice (the partner or spouse, the only child, the nearest relative, the best friend) or, with no one else around, how could they desert the patient in a time of need?

Many people fall into caregiving by accident. They want to help, they feel obligated to help, or a little of both. They may have natural fears about their own futures, such as how they will be cared for or how their children will be cared for. They may do someone a "favor" in hopes that it will be returned if and when they need it themselves.

Regardless of the reason for doing it, if you're reading this book, you're proactive about being a compassionate, effective caregiver. You want to go into this with your eyes open and a little mental preparation will go a long way. With some introspection, you will be able to answer these questions about your own situation.

What Do I Say? Questions For Yourself About Caregiving

- How involved do I want to be? Do I want to take this on full-time or part-time, regularly or occasionally?

- What can I manage physically for the patient, without inflicting injury to myself? Do I have constraints that may limit my ability to get the patient what she needs? (For example: Are you fighting a serious illness, pregnant, or medically fragile?)

- What can I manage emotionally without feeling resentful? Can I allow myself to care for and love someone that may not have the ability to thank me? Can I step up to being the parent to my parent or to being the head of my household?

- What can I manage financially without putting myself in jeopardy? Do I have the capacity to take over medical costs, if needed?

- Will I be able to juggle my life and her care? Can I take on increased responsibilities, not just from taking care of patient, but taking over her role(s) as well?

- How much can I rationally discuss with the patient?

- If I change my decision to give care, is there someone who can take my place? Who is it?

Even a tentative response to these questions will get you headed in the right direction on your caregiver journey. Thinking through the questions may be tough but it's worth the time. When you've done so, congratulate yourself for taking the next steps. You may have a long way to travel, so let's get your approach in order.

Setting Up for Success

"Some caregivers are compared to Mother Teresa," says Wanda, 48, who cares for her father with pancreatic cancer. "Me, I'm more like Sally Field in 'The Flying Nun' or Julie Andrews in 'The Sound of Music.' I'll get things done, but maybe not in the conventional way."

Because each patient situation is different, there are no cookie cutter approaches to caregiving. However, there are ways to set yourself up for a successful experience. The idea is to facilitate good care to the patient while limiting the negative impacts to you.

You can achieve this by following three simple steps:

Step 1:   Determine what being a "good" caregiver means to you.

Step 2:   Lay the groundwork for communicating with the patient.

Step 3:   Empower the patient to take part in his healing.

Let's take a look at what each of these means.

Step 1:   Determine What Being a "Good" Caregiver Means To You.

> *"There's so much information out there about cancer and being with a cancer patient. I'm not sure what to believe," says Walt, 48. "How can I find out the best way to go? Or what applies to me and my son? We have so many questions."*

What do you expect from yourself? Your expectations will form a framework in which you will make choices about what you do for the patient and for yourself. You will also make assessments about how well you're doing these things.

Perhaps you can start with expectations like this:

"Being a good caregiver means that I will listen to the patient and support him. I will address his reasonable needs in accordance with medical advice. I will be able to show tough love when it's in his best interest. I know I can get assistance if something is harmful to me or if I am medically or physically unable to do it. I will take time for myself to keep my own health up while the patient is on the mend."

Think about it. Add or subtract words to the expectations so they make sense for your situation. Give yourself permission not to be "perfect" by others' standards or "accessible 24x7." Allow yourself to do things for you. Give others the opportunity to help you to be the best caregiver you can be, according to what it means to you.

Step 2: Lay the groundwork for positive interactions and conversations with the patient.

"Why do I feel like he's yelling at me?" says Vanessa, 66, whose father is fighting melanoma. "I'm trying to help him."

You may need some additional ideas about interacting with the patient. No one can expect to go through this kind of experience without changes to an existing relationship.

Most patients will experience emotional traumas and practical difficulties, which means there will be a roller coaster of reactions. These may last days, months, or even years. Even if the patient is normally pretty consistent, dealing with a serious disease will place him off-kilter for a while. So plan for the storm – you could be in for some inclement weather.

Your weighty job IS NOT to help the patient accept that he has cancer. That will happen (or not) in his own time. Your job IS to be ready, if and when he accepts this and wants to express it. Heed the advice of other caregivers and "thicken your skin." When dealing with your own reactions to the DIAGNOSIS (see glossary for explanation of terms in small caps), you will be challenged to deal with his anger, his anxiety, his depression, or other reactions. Your strength and patience will be tested: Being the primary caregiver, you will likely bear the brunt of those reactions simply because of your proximity. If you try to remain rational, it could help avoid a misunderstanding that could damage your relationship.

These suggestions may prove useful when interacting with the patient:

- Be flexible. Regardless of how well you know the patient, your best approach is to be ready to adapt to changing circumstances. If you're rigid, it can lead to friction with the patient and to internal stress for you.

- Let the patient direct his life. Help him accomplish what he wants, the way he wants. Ask if his activities are things he can do himself and, if so, let him do them. Don't do it for him.

- Find ways to celebrate in the midst of the illness. Recognize anniversaries, holidays, or birthdays with good conversation, music, and relaxation. Do things that are unrelated to cancer. Do things you both want to do, not just activities that are good for him.

Whatever the situation, try to maneuver it so that it becomes an opportunity for you to get to know the patient better or to understand his source of frustration. When you interact with the patient, you may discover that the effects of what you say can be long lasting. The section that follows provides some tips on how to manage conversations with the patient.

What Do I Say? Talking with the Patient

It's tough to know when to bring difficult topics out in the open. It can be emotionally painful for both of you to talk about the disease or its effects.

There will probably be times when simply being with the patient (without words) works best. During those times, you can support him with your presence and your comforting nods. Trust your instinct on what's best and do it.

For times when the patient seems to want to talk, consider these recommendations:

- Start by asking him if this is a good time to visit. Ask if he wants some company or if he would like some time to himself.

- The patient may need some encouragement to start. Try using phrases like: "We can talk about your diagnosis. Cancer's not a bad word. Almost everyone has been touched by it in one way or another. We'll figure out what to do. We can get through this and we will."

- Encourage honest communications between the two of you. Be truthful but not hurtful and don't be afraid to tell him your needs to such as: "We both need our strength. Let's get some rest."

- Build the patient's confidence and self-esteem by complimenting him when you can and being supportive of what he does on his own.

- Use the time together to discuss problems and possible solutions.

- Keep the conversation to a healthy length, usually no more than two hours at a time. If you need to cut it short, say something like: "Let's continue this tomorrow, when we have more time."

It's important to remember that the patient needs to be involved in the decision-making process about his own care. When it's time to make a decision, begin by telling him the situation and outlining the options. Let him make the choice and follow through with whatever he chooses to do.

Step 3: Empower the Patient to Take Part in His Healing

"It's like his cancer diagnosis came with a license to be a couch potato," says Pam, 32. "My boyfriend needs to figure out that I may not be here all the time to wait on him. Why doesn't he do more for himself?"

One of the most difficult challenges in caregiving is knowing what the patient can do for himself. As the disease and the treatment progress, the patient will have different sensitivities and constraints on his abilities. It's up to you to watch for verbal and non-verbal cues. These can help you to recognize those things that the patient is capable of on his own, with a little encouragement or guidance, and what he absolutely cannot do.

Usually, the patient has the capability to educate himself about the disease and possible courses of treatment. In addition to the materials given to him by his medical professionals, he can read books, articles in newspapers, or information on the internet. He can start to understand how some of his current negative habits (like smoking, excessive drinking or eating) can influence his condition and how to change those things if he chooses to do so. He can also learn what his options are in terms of traditional treatments, non-traditional treatments and CLINICAL TRIALS. The more he knows, the better he will be able to make upcoming decisions and increase the likelihood of attaining treatment goals.

As his caregiver, be determined that he take an active part in what needs to be done to encourage his own healing. Like Pam in the quote above, you'll want to see him doing what he can to fight the disease. Empower him through supporting his efforts and by getting him the information he needs. Let him take it from there.

Constructive, honest exchanges with the patient will round out the actions you can take to set yourself up for a successful caregiving experience. They will also enhance the opportunity for a positive outcome for the patient. Keep up the good work, but don't forget to take care of yourself, too.

Taking Care of Yourself

> *"Take care of myself? Who are you kidding," says Sewellen, 44, whose daughter is fighting leukemia. "How would that look? I'll keep my hair appointments and everything else will have to wait."*

We're about to let you in on a closely guarded secret. The Number One Rule of Caregiving is this: "You must maintain an even balance between the patient's concerns and your personal concerns."

In other words, you can't give good care if you're in bad shape yourself. Complement the efforts to make her well by maintaining your own health. This means you need to make sure your health is in good standing. If you have health concerns yourself, address them in relation to her care. Be mindful of your own nutrition. Get exercise and rest, whenever you can.

It's important to be kind to yourself mentally, too. Most likely, you are not a professional caregiver. Don't beat yourself up for not knowing what to do or say. You'll find a way to make it through the tough times. Don't berate yourself for being emotional. Whatever you're feeling is OK. Don't assume you're just stupid if you're having a hard time understanding medical information. It takes a lot of effort to listen and to digest new information. You're doing great so far.

Your own support network can help validate your feelings and help you deal with a variety of issues that surface. If you can, identify two or three people outside any existing family to form your network. Make it a point to see or to call each person, just to keep in touch. You'll build the patient's support network later, but you need to be sustained in the meantime.

Staying in touch with members of your support network can help safeguard you from depression. Depression is more than feeling down for a few days – it's a force that can be debilitating for you. In addition to sadness and fatigue, depression can bring you difficulty with sleeping, eating, concentrating, and meeting responsibilities. It's common to fight these symptoms when your're faced with lifestyle adjustments, illness, and changing relationships.

Give yourself permission to be sad and to grieve, but be aware that when the sadness and other symptoms continue for weeks on end, it's time to lean on others. Talking to your friends or to trained professionals about the issues may be the best (but not necessarily the easiest!) way to acknowledge them and work towards a solution. Therapists, doctors, social workers, and spiritual leadres (like chaplains, rabbis, or ministers) are trained to offer you guidance on your situation. Some of these offer their services for free while others may charge for their time, but it may well be worth your investment in mental health.

Most importantly, remember that you're not alone. Being a caregiver can be isolating and consuming. If you are unsure of how to build a network or if you want private guidance and support, consider seeing a therapist, a minister, or another counselor. Giving care is most likely a new role for you and you may have to deal with a lot of changes. Take heart: Others have gone through this experience and they've made it through successfully. You will, too.

Wrapping Up

Both you and the patient will be changed by this experience with a serious illness. As you've read this chapter, you have been presented with a lot to think about in terms of your new position as a caregiver and the lifestyle impacts that can accompany it. You now have a better understanding of the roles you may be asked to play and you've made decisions about what your involvement in the patient's care will be.

You've just started your journey as a more informed, better prepared caregiver. Be sure to concentrate on the road ahead but remember these steps:

- Act according to what being a "good" caregiver means to you, not what it might mean to anyone else.

- Initiate positive interactions and helpful dialogue with the patient.

- Encourage the patient to take an active part in her healing.

- Keep an even balance between the patient's concerns and your personal concerns.

It's also important to understand the patient's perspective. In the next chapter, we will talk about the patient's MEDICAL HISTORY, her present needs, and the next steps.

Chapter 2: Knowing the Patient

"I've learned more about my cousin in these past couple of months than in all the rest of our years," says Laura, 44. "Going to the doctor's office to treat her ovarian cancer has opened my eyes to who she is as a person, medically and non-medically."

You've begun to learn about the caregiving responsibilities and their potential personal impacts. Now it's time to really get to know the patient.

You may think you know the patient as a spouse/partner, a relative, or a friend. You may be able to anticipate what she might normally do. However, illnesses often impact a personality or reveal aspects of a personality that are normally "hidden." As circumstances demand more of the patient, those changes may become visible in terms of relationships, priorities, and attitudes. Like Laura in the quote above, you may discover parts of the patient you've never encountered.

When you take on the role of caregiver, you may also take on the role of decision-maker on issues that have major impacts on both of your lives. If you understand the patient's personality and wishes for care, it may smooth the way in upcoming decision-making. You will want to think through the choices yourself and know (through discussion and documentation) the patient's requests and opinions.

The goal of this chapter is to formalize the patient's wishes for care. To help you begin, we will describe:

- What You Need to Know About the Patient's Personal and MEDICAL HISTORY

- Personal Documents (Business and Medical Planning)

- ADVANCE DIRECTIVE DOCUMENTS that Reflect Wishes for Future Treatment

- How to Discuss Sensitive Subjects and Make Decisions with the Patient

- Ways to Take Care of Yourself.

The more you know, the more effective you can be. You may not be confronted with all of the disease-related issues for which you have prepared but, as the saying goes, "an ounce of prevention is worth a pound of cure." Gathering this information can also help you become the patient advocate who interacts with the patient's medical professionals. We'll start by talking about what that means.

Being the Patient's Advocate

"My mom asked me to speak for him when he can't speak for himself," says Indie, 50, whose father is fighting tongue and throat cancers. "I don't know what that entails but shouldn't he ask me that?"

In the last chapter, we mentioned that part of being a caregiver to a cancer patient is being his advocate to medical professionals. When you're with the patient in a medical setting, you will meet and talk with people that need information about the patient so that he will get the care he needs. You will begin to have a relationship with these professionals and have question-and-answer exchanges with them about the patient.

Being a patient advocate means being able to accurately speak about the patient's situation and his needs. You may be an advocate when the patient can speak for himself and when he can't. Knowing information about three areas of the patient's life will help you appropriately represent the patient. These three areas are: the patient's medical background (past), what's happening with him now (present), and what he would like in terms of future care (future). Let's discuss each one.

Reviewing Their Past

"That was years ago. She's healed from that," says Carl, 77, of his wife's prior diagnosis of colon cancer. "Why does that matter now?"

Whether you want to revisit it or not, the patient's past is important. Sometimes, especially with a prior DIAGNOSIS, it can be painful to review a person's history. However, an understanding of her medical and personal history helps the medical professionals:

- Determine the approach to care

- Deal with hereditary factors

- Anticipate possible complications

- Estimate the PROGNOSIS.

It's important that you, the patient, and the healthcare professionals share information. Establish your relationship to the patient and inform the others about the patient's history. As caregiver, you will want to be informed of the patient's condition, her prognosis, and her special needs. Be aware that you may not have access to this data unless you have been given permission by the patient, because of recent legislation.

In April of 1996, Congress instituted the Health Insurance Portability and Accountability Act, otherwise known as HIPAA. Designed to protect the confidentiality of patient health information, HIPAA restricts the release of information to anyone except the patient, unless the patient signs away that right. It also recommends that a patient should only disclose personal information to a family member, friend, or other person to help with individual healthcare or healthcare payments.

Advocates of HIPAA say it is important for the patient to know that her personal information is secure and it will not be shared without permission. Therefore, if you need to be involved in care planning and treatment, be sure to work with the patient to include your name on all HIPAA forms and keep a copy of the authorization with you. If not, you will not have access to relevant information and you may not be invited to consultations or office visits.

The first thing you do in most doctors' offices is fill out HIPAA and health history forms. You or the patient will need to know and clearly answer questions on standard medical health history, including:

1. What is the chief complaint? What symptoms is the patient having that the healthcare professionals need to know about? When did they start? How have they changed?

2. What healthcare coverage does the patient have (private, group, Medicare, none)?

3. Is any kind of cancer present in the patient's medical history or the family's medical history?

4. What other health problems/considerations does the patient have? What previous treatments (like CHEMOTHERAPY and surgery) has the patient had and when? Does the patient have any allergies?

5. What medications (prescription and otherwise) is the patient taking? What complementary/alternative therapies has the patient tried or does the patient continue to use?

6. Who are the other doctors involved in the patient's care?

7. What is the patient's work history?

8. What are the patient's habits in terms of eating, exercise, alcohol, and cigarette use?

With a cancer diagnosis, you'll likely deal with multiple specialists in various settings. Each one will want to know about the patient's past. You may want to write the answers down and carry them with you, so that you provide consistent information to everyone. This could be significant in understanding the patient's present situation.

Understanding Their Present

*"I never thought my grandfather would give up smoking,"
said Marie, 40. "Even when I was a little girl, I remember
him having fancy pipes and cigars. He smoked for decades
and loved it. But when the doctor said it was lung cancer, he
quit 'cold turkey.'"*

Most caregivers are close to or related to their patients. Often, they
know the patient's habits and can correctly estimate the patient's
decisions. They may understand the patient's personality and response
to regular stresses. But the diagnosis of a serious disease has the
power to change patient attitudes, beliefs, and even routines.

Knowing the patient's present needs and watching for his reactions will
help you manage current situations. Ask yourself (and when possible,
the patient) a few questions: "What is his need for information about
the illness, treatment, and prognosis?" "What is his need for social
interaction or solitude?" "What is his way of communicating with
me?"

You'll discover many of his needs from his reactions. Ask the patient
how this diagnosis is affecting him. Or, just watch his behavior for
a while. Pay attention to how he responds to medical instructions.
Notice how his routine changes. Make a mental note of the times
when he wants to talk about the illness.

Your observations and your discussions will affect how you interact
with the patient on a daily basis. When you share this information
with the healthcare professionals, it plays a key part in planning the
patient's future care.

Thinking About Their Future

"You hear about those families arguing on T.V.," says Arnold, 25. "My mom says we're not doing that with our uncle. We're making decisions now, just in case he doesn't beat this esophageal cancer and needs life support."

If you know the patient's past and current situation, it can help you identify important future care issues to address with the patient. Directly asking – and honestly answering – specific questions helps to ensure that future care is administered according to the patient's wishes. If you understand the patient's wishes, you can comfort and reassure him through confident decision-making.

If the time comes when you need answers to important treatment or end-of-life questions, you will want to have the patient's requests and opinions in writing. When Advanced Directive documents are discussed, completed, and filed:

- You will have less "guesswork" and fewer agonizing decisions to make because they've already been made. You'll also avoid the emotionally-charged situation of: "I don't know…We never talked about it."

- You will reduce the possibility of arguing with others about treatment decisions.

- You can eliminate the worry if you've forgotten something or the guilt if you remember it later.

Putting these ADVANCE DIRECTIVE DOCUMENTS in place is a good measure to take regardless of health history and current condition and it can never be harmful. It may, however, require some skilled "maneuvers" and discussions. Later in the chapter, you will read some suggestions on approaching this decision-making as a dance.

The manner in which Advanced Directive documents are drafted, executed, and enforced varies per state. As this is an evolving area of law, changes to laws that govern these may happen day to day. Their general intentions are further discussed in the next sections.

Planning Documents

Finding out what you need to know is a great place to begin when working with the patient to identify his needs. It's often helpful to have pre-printed lists or forms so you don't miss any essential items.

The two parts that follow divide the recommended data into personal documents and medical documents. These are only guidelines; you may want to get additional advice from an attorney, a tax accountant, a financial advisor, or an estate planner. You may want to record only what makes sense for your situation. You might also consider local law requirements – there may be different "validity" standards, such as the need to have witnesses or a notary present.

As you work on this, don't forget to congratulate yourself on getting to this stage – it's often difficult to discuss these issues and whatever decisions you are able to make and whatever you are able to document will be helpful to you in the future.

Personal Documentation

Both you and the patient should have copies of (or ready access to) family and personal papers. Usually, the issuing entity will be able to make available whatever paperwork you need, provided that you are able to give them proof of identity and intent.

The next table includes recommendations on which vital records, financial data, and business/work-related information you should secure. These are usually very straightforward and often have the title of the document on the front (at the very top). Depending on the complexity of your situation, you may identify more forms or papers that would be necessary to have at hand when needed and you should include copies of those as well. Try to put together as much as possible and never worry that you have too many papers together: better to have too many than to have information missing.

Personal Business Documents

List of Documents	Who to Contact
Birth and marriage certificates	Bureau of Vital Statistics
Burial plans	Patient, friend, or family member
Business-related documents, especially for small business owners: operations records, partnership agreements, buy/sell agreements with partners, insurance, limited partnerships to specify transfer of wealth in a company	Business owners, investors
Eligibility for civil service benefits	Department of employment
Employee benefits or pension plans	Company of employment
Family trust information	Estate planner, financial advisor
Insurance information: policy numbers, terms, beneficiaries	Insurance company
List of family, friends, significant people	Patient, friend, family member
List of liabilities (mortgages, personal or business loans, car notes, credit cards, school loans)	Patient, friend, family member, issuing lenders
List of property or assets (land, jewelry, furniture)	County government (property), insurance company
Military benefits	Military Benefits Counselor (Army, Navy, Air Force, Marines, Coast Guard), Veteran's Administration
Rough draft of obituary	Patient, friend, family member
Social Security benefits	Social Security Administration
Tax returns	Internal Revenue Service
Will	Patient or attorney

When you're thinking about other financial/estate matters, discuss treatment and other care as well. You and the patient have the right to make choices and decisions – based on an understanding of the patient's illness – and the right to have those decisions respected. The next section addresses specific medical documentation and your right to specify your wishes.

Medical Documentation

Health-related planning documents can be confusing. The differences between the documents may be unclear and you may wonder why you and the patient would need them in the first place.

You can avoid some of the questions and the confusion by completing Advance Directive documents. ADVANCE (ahead of time) DIRECTIVE (direction or guidance) documents capture the patient's wishes for providing or withholding treatment – both at the beginning and throughout the course of illness or injury. The information in these documents applies to a wide range of possible situations, from car accidents to life-limiting illness. Advance Directive documents enable doctors, family, and other caregivers to know what treatment a person would want, in the event that he is unable to speak for himself. It's critical that you not only understand what documents are available to you, but that you also understand what issues they address. Descriptions of widely-recognized documents are given in the sections that follow.

The two major pieces of the Advance Directive documents are the *Healthcare Power of Attorney* and the *Living Will*. These two documents may be separate or combined. While the rules surrounding these documents vary by state, they generally:

- Take effect only when a patient is unable to make decisions

- Should be used with medical recommendations on current situation

- Do not require a lawyer to draft in most states, do not apply to financial affairs, and may be updated at any time prior to incapacitation.

These Advance Directive documents are important and while they may not be used in their entirety, they should be completed to the best of the patient's ability. If these informed choices are made, the healthcare professionals will honor the patient's wishes and give care accordingly. In the absence of Advance Directive documents, the professionals will continue to treat the patient until they are told to stop by the family (following the legal succession for blood relatives: spouse, children, parents, siblings) or by the caregiver.

Healthcare Power of Attorney

The Healthcare Power of Attorney document simply *appoints a particular person* to make medical decisions for the person who can no longer make them for himself. This document is also called a Healthcare Proxy, an Appointment of a Healthcare Agent, or a Durable Power of Attorney for Health Care. It differs from a Durable Power of Attorney because it applies only to making decisions on medical care (as opposed to legal matters) when the patient is physically incapacitated and cannot make them alone. The person appointed may be called a healthcare agent, surrogate, attorney-in-fact, or healthcare proxy. When we refer to the Power of Attorney, we are talking about the person who has that right or that responsibility.

Power of Attorney documents are separate because many people want a different person making their healthcare decisions than the one making their financial decisions. Additionally, the person granted this power for the patient may also be different from the designated family spokesperson, who may have opinions on the patient's care that differ from the patient's requests. With that document in place, the patient is still in control, through his appointed person. If no other person is granted Power of Attorney, the healthcare professionals will make the decision for the patient.

Will

There are two types of wills: a Traditional Will and a Living Will. It is important to understand that Traditional Wills are NOT medical documents.

Traditional Wills address distribution of property and other personal items after the owner has died. They answer the question "What do I want them to do with my money/belongings after I'm gone?" Traditional Wills can be filed at a probate court and an attorney may serve as the custodian. Burial wishes are sometimes included.

If a person has not drafted it at the time of his death (which is called "dying intestate"), most states will furnish a Traditional Will but it may not be consistent with his wishes. Many people think that if they have completed a Last Will and Testament, their healthcare wishes are covered – which is NOT true because this is a Traditional Will and it only covers belongings.

Living Wills outline which treatments the patient wants or does not want at the end of his life. They are meant to guide family and doctors in deciding how aggressively to use medical treatments intended to prolong the process of dying. A Living Will is also called Healthcare Declaration or Medical Directive.

Living Wills do not deal with property or other possessions. Instead, they include treatment information regarding:

- Do Not Resuscitate (DNR) – Does he want efforts to revive him if he stops breathing or his heart stops beating? Unless the patient has signed a DNR Order that directs healthcare professionals not to apply cardiopulmonary resuscitation (CPR) or begin mechanical ventilation, every effort will be made to resuscitate him.

- Life Sustaining Treatments – Would he want efforts to prolong his life? Life sustaining treatments (LST) replace or support an essential bodily function and they are intended to prolong the process of dying. Unless there are orders in place, these will be administered by medical professionals when necessary. They include:

  o Breathing Assistance and CPR (covered under a DNR order). The patient may become a candidate for CPR, mechanical ventilation, or INTUBATION if he is having trouble breathing, his breathing has stopped, or his heart has stopped.

  o Artificial Hydration and Nutrition. When a patient becomes unable to eat or drink by mouth, he may be a candidate for artificial nutrition and hydration through a tube to sustain life. Sometimes referred to as "tube-feeding," artificial nutrition and hydration provide food and fluids through either a tube down the nose into the stomach, a tube directly into the stomach, or an IV into a vein to sustain life.

  o Dialysis. Multiple methods exist to substitute for the kidneys cleansing the blood to remove toxins.

  o Antibiotics. Some medical professionals believe that administering these drugs is necessary to combat additional serious infections, such as pneumonia. Others believe that using antibiotics prolong unnecessary suffering.

- Blood Transfusions – Would he agree to receive blood as a means of sustaining his life? Some spiritual practices limit the transfer of blood or blood components from one person to another.

- Pain Management – Would he agree to medication to control his pain even if it may be addictive or speed up his own death? Pain may be present when the disease follows its normal course; minimizing that pain is always important, particularly if the pain is crippling.

- Do Not Hospitalize (DNH) – Most patients prefer to die at home. If he is a nursing home resident or ill at home, should he be transported to the hospital for care, risking problems in transportation? Is it time to shift the treatment goal from cure to comfort care only?

- Organ Donation – Would he be interested in donating a part of his body for use by another or for scientific teaching? Many people do not realize that more than 20 kinds of organs and tissues can be donated, including: heart, liver, lungs, kidneys, pancreas, small intestine, corneas, bone, heart valves, and skin.

- Cremation and religious customs – Does he have some special rituals or needs? Most documents have space to write down other specific requests.

In many states, any form of Living Will will be sufficient – even the proverbial "napkin" – as long as it's signed. In other states, such as Maryland, only a formal document that has been notarized will be recognized. Again, if a person dies without a Living Will in place, the medical professionals will continue to treat the patient until they are told to stop by the family (following the legal succession for blood relatives: spouse, children, parents, siblings) or by the caregiver.

With a serious illness like cancer, there are other items to consider while putting the Advance Directive documents in place, such as gene therapy or other CLINICAL TRIALS. The basic questions are:

- Would he be interested in learning about current research with his particular kind of cancer?

- How does he feel about furthering this research?

- Would he consider participation in clinical trials where the outcome is uncertain?

Generally, young and otherwise healthy individuals are more interested in and more encouraged to participate in these than elderly patients with multiple health issues. Keep in mind, his opinion or desires may change if the situation becomes more pressing.

What Do I Say? Interacting with the Patient

Few people are comfortable talking about the possibilities of life-challenging situations with a patient who needs to discuss this. If you're in a supporting role, you may be uncomfortable as well. Try to be a good listener and limit your own opinions. Remember that this may *affect* you, but it's not *about* you. There are no right or wrong answers.

A series of bigger questions exist at the core of the Advance Directive documents:

- How much are we going to push to keep the patient living?

- How long should life be supported – hours, days, months, years?

- If he is dying anyway, why even start life sustaining treatments?

These are serious value judgments to be made and thinking is not usually clear during a crisis. A good start is to secure an Advance Directive document to help you organize the discussion and to clarify the next steps. Because it formally outlines requests from the patient, the document decreases the amount of emotional impact in making these decisions. When possible, allow enough time to carefully consider all questions and to review all options. You can avoid personal errors in judgments or family disputes by documenting these things before a crisis occurs.

The important thing in talking about these sensitive subjects is to be compassionate with the patient. Some caregivers will be able to think of just the right words to say because they know the patient so well. You may have several unsuccessful attempts at having them listen to your questions but keep trying. This will benefit both of you.

Here are some questions and phrases to get you talking:

- I care about you. We need to make sure that I know what you want to have happen in certain situations.

- We need to have a plan. How can you be sure that your wishes are honored if we don't know what they are?

- Are you reluctant to talk about this? Are you scared?

- I found this document, which I think can help us. We can talk about what it says. Is that OK?

- Things are harder to do at the last minute. I think we can prepare using this document. If we choose to complete this, it can be changed at any time.

- Are you concerned with pain management?

- What religious concerns or end-of-life customs do you have that I need to be aware of?

- Are you thinking about how money may play a part in your decisions of care?

- Is there someone else you would like to be involved in this planning process? If not me, who do we call in case of emergency, who will know your wishes and will be able to speak for you, if you cannot?

If the patient won't complete a pre-printed form, try to get him to answer some of the questions. Even if you get only general answers, you can write them down and, if the time comes, the entire burden of decision-making will not rest with you.

Decision-Making as a Dance

"My aunt always made the decisions around here," says Tom, 30. "I guess that's because she raised me. But she doesn't like talking about treatment stuff. I guess she figures we'll all have to deal with it later."

At the beginning of the caregiving process, it's critical to establish the relationship and the roles that you have with the patient. Often, that relationship is already in place, such as mother-daughter, husband-wife/partner-partner or aunt-nephew, as in the quote above. It sets the stage for communication and action.

Roles will change during the course of the illness. For example, a mother who has guided her daughter through the years may suddenly find that she needs the daughter to guide her healthcare decisions, treatments, and routine. This can be extremely taxing on both parties, especially if there is reluctance on either side to do so.

The patient and other family members may not want to complete or even talk about future planning of any kind, much less health-related subjects, for any number of reasons. You may not want to talk about treatment or end-of-life issues either. But holding these discussions and making decisions on these topics is necessary – in fact, these can be *the most critical decisions of a person's life.* As caregiver, you need to take the lead on having these discussions and documenting the patient's needs – after all, this will affect you too.

It may be helpful to think of the decision-making process as a dance. Everyone has her own style, but the idea is to try to move in sync, even if it takes a little practice. To some people, this will come naturally and smoothly. To others, this will be clumsy, creating potentially hurtful results. As you change your movements, your "dance partner" (the patient) will change as well. You'll find that the more you communicate, the better your dance will be.

Here's an example:

Knowing the Patient

Dance of Decision-Making

You, The Caregiver...	Interact With the Patient By...
Decide to get in the dance. You decide to start planning future health care.	Gathering background information or documents that will help you organize your discussion. Plan to spend at least an hour talking.
Ask the patient to dance. You begin a conversation about Advance Directive documents.	Being in a place where it's easy to talk and approach the patient. It may be more comfortable to have someone else join you. Maybe a chaplain, social worker, or other spiritual leader could participate in the conversation.
Encounter a little uncertainty and resistance.	Thinking up possible objectives and solutions and sharing them with the patient.
Lead them to the dance floor. You provide them with a list of questions or documents.	Encouraging the patient to talk about these subjects and permitting them to lead in pace and direction. Remember that the patient's wishes should lead the healthcare course.
Take your stance. You tell them your understanding of the healthcare decision.	Recording as much of the details as possible. Perhaps you can fill out your paperwork as the patient fills out her paperwork.
Dance together. Both the caregiver and patient contribute to the conversation. There must be input/yield on either side.	Being mindful not to "step on her toes" if she thinks you're trying to influence or push her in any way. Adjust your style to match hers but don't be afraid to ask her to modify her approach as well. You'll both be less bruised for it.
Pirouette and try new moves. You discuss options that may be frightening.	Repeating the process if you encounter more resistance and have to stop mid-dance.

You, The Caregiver...	Interact With the Patient By...
Finish the dance. You complete the documents or the discussion.	Thanking each other and consider more dancing (decision-making) if the time is right.
Go back to your seat. You follow through on filing the documents and placing copies where they need to be.	Letting her know that her wishes will be carried out. She is probably tired but glad she got up for "the dance."

At times, it will be difficult for the caregiver to respect the patient's wishes or for the patient to respect the caregiver's other responsibilities or constraints. For this dance to be successful, one person should be leading and the other following. While the patient's wishes will guide the direction of the dance, it is the caregiver who leads the "moves" in the process to support those wishes.

If the decision-making process comes to a standstill, the medical professionals can give guidance on issues, but resulting actions are ultimately up to the patient or to the person designated as the Healthcare Power of Attorney. The next section provides some ideas on overcoming objections with the patient.

What Do I Say? Overcoming Objections to Documenting Advance Directives

Here are some common objections to completing Advance Directive documents, as well as some ideas on how to respond.

- **What are these documents? Why do we need to do this?** Tell her that you want to be sure that her voice is heard and that her wishes are known and respected. Talk about advances in modern medicine that can keep her alive for weeks, months, or even years.

- **We don't even know how serious this illness is.** This will help both the caregiver and the patient know what care the patient wants to receive if it becomes necessary.

- **I have seen similar situations on TV and I don't want to drag the family through anything like that.** Exactly. Situations happen like this in the hospital every day. They are not announced to the public when the affairs are in order.

- **I've taken care of myself my whole life. I don't want to burden others or ask for help.** She may or may not say this directly. Maybe she does not know how to ask for help and needs to be encouraged to do so. In either case, it can be a sticky situation. Try to go at her pace and plan as much as you can. You need her cooperation, however, and you may have to tell her that directly.

- **I'm pregnant. What if one of these treatments endangers my healthy pregnancy or the baby's birth?** If the woman is pregnant and a cancer patient or hoping to conceive post-treatment, she is already facing serious decisions for herself and her child. It is critical that she works with her medical professionals as soon as possible to complete the Advance Directive documents.

- **I have no money to pay for any of these treatments so I just won't have any of them.** Explain that these treatments do cost money, but that some of them are covered by Medicare, Medicaid, or insurance. Even without insurance coverage, the treatments will automatically be given in a crisis situation, unless there are express instructions not to do so. In that case, the bill for services will be sent to the family for payment.

- **I will fill them out for the children, but not for myself.** If the parent has custody of the children, it is important that she is taken care of first, so that her children do not have to worry about being part of the decision or making the decision themselves (provided they are of legal age).

- **I don't want to 'bother' doctors or nurses unless the emergency is happening. They'll know what to do.** Unless you have recorded `your wishes, they will *not* know what the patient would like them to do. Administering care is their job and if you have special considerations, they need to know them.

- **If I talk about things like that, I'll just be 'tempting fate' and cause these problems (or death) to happen.** This is just a precautionary measure. You may not be faced with these issues now but it's best to be prepared, especially if you have personal beliefs against the administration of life support/life sustaining treatments. They will be complete for future use, whenever that may be.

Documenting the Patient's Wishes

"Once we had a printed document, I proceeded to ask him questions as if it were just another form from the doctor's office," says Joshua, 48. "He answered everything directly."

By now, you've probably started a conversation with the patient regarding future planning. If you've been able to talk through issues to the point where you are able to make decisions, the next question is: How do make sure I have covered everything and how do I document it?

Fortunately, there is a wide range of helpful pre-printed documents that you may order by mail and download from the internet that will guide you. In preparing for treatment issues, you will want to be sure that you give careful consideration to all issues.

See the Resource Directory in the back of this book for web sites that may assist in future care planning. If you're unsure about specific requirements for your state, hire an attorney who handles such matters to help you through the process.

How Can I Help? Finding Sample Forms and Documents

Helping the patient secure and complete documents relaying his wishes – his Advance Directive documents – may be difficult at first, but it will provide peace of mind if needed in the future.

It is relatively easy to find these documents. Many varieties exist because they are not federally regulated. As you begin to look, you will see the volume of options available, which can be overwhelming to both of you. Try to keep it basic and search for forms that address these decisions:

- Healthcare Power of Attorney – Who does he want to make decisions about his care when he can't make them for himself?

- Do Not Resuscitate (DNR) Order – Does he want efforts to revive him if he stops breathing or if his heart stops beating?

- Life Sustaining Treatments – Would he want efforts to prolong his life, including:

  o Breathing Assistance and CPR (covered under a DNR order)

  o Hydration and Nutrition

  o Dialysis

  o Antibiotics

- Blood Transfusions – Would he agree to receive blood as a means of sustaining his life?

- Pain Management – Would he agree to medication to control his pain even if it may speed up his own death?

- Hospitalization, organ donation, cremation, religious customs, and where he would like to die, if possible.

You may need to spend some time searching for the right document. Civic and volunteer organizations for seniors, community centers, and hospitals provide information for healthcare planning. Some attorneys can provide you with suggestions for Advance Directive documents or you may be interested in focusing your search online. If so, try web sites on Living Wills and other Advance Directive documents to narrow your search results.

Completing and Filing the Forms

"We did it," says Niko, 60, whose wife is fighting gastric cancer. "First ones in my family for generations. Now all our children will see the importance and fill out these documents."

After you have secured a document that you are both comfortable with, read through it. Be thorough and try not to rush. Take the time needed to discuss each issue and to write it down exactly the way you both want it. Be firm but loving.

Complete each section, even if it does not apply to the patient. For example, if the patient is unmarried, write "not applicable" in spaces asking for spousal information. You'll want to discuss all the issues covered in these documents and write your wishes down appropriately. If you haven't addressed a certain topic and it arises, you may be rushed in your decisions. The patient's medical professionals can guide you on these issues, but resulting actions are ultimately up to the patient or to the person granted Power Of Attorney.

If you have the luxury of putting the document away for a few days and then reviewing it at a later time, take that opportunity. The more precise you can be now, the clearer everyone who uses the document in the future will be.

Most forms require a witness or two; some states require a notary or lawyer to be present during completion or at least to review the document's contents. After you have completed the form, research how it needs to be acknowledged and filed. Think carefully how you will share Advance Directive documents with others. As painful or awkward as it may be, it is the most effective way to ensure that the patient's wishes are followed. At the very minimum, inform a family member or friend that the patient's requests are recorded and the location where a copy can be found.

As you assist the patient in completing her Advance Directive documents, be sure to place a copy in an easy-to-find place in the home. You'll be able to locate it quickly when you need it.

After you've completed and filed the patient's Advance Directive documents, share them with the medical professionals. Then they will be informed of the patient's needs and they can facilitate care according to documented requests. You can do this by bringing a copy of a formal Advance Directive document to your doctor's office. Provide revisions to them if your needs change over time.

It's sometimes challenging to determine what is medically relevant or significant – that is, what and how much to tell the medical professionals involved in the patient's care. While they may want to listen, they are often stretched with multiple patients. To ensure that they have the time to see them all, they must be careful how much time they spend with each one.

Most of the physicians interviewed for this book agreed that patients and caregivers should err on the side of being prepared to tell detailed information but to stay on the subject of what is asked. This may mean that the doctor does not know every detail, but he may not need every detail. Use the questions mentioned earlier in this chapter as a guide. Your precise answers to address what he is asking will help the physician make quicker and better assessments.

What Do I Say: Talking to Others

Talking to medical professionals may be much easier than talking to non-professionals who may be curious about how and why you are choosing to document your Advance Directive documents. After people hear that you are involved in this process, several common questions may surface. It may be that they are interested in doing this for themselves and they want to learn more about it. They may just want to know specifics about your situation. It may be some combination of the two.

Whatever the case, don't be compelled to give particulars to them if you don't want to share. Instead, give them a blank copy of an Advance Directive document that you're completing or refer them to a helpful web site. But if you do want to answer them, here are some ideas. Don't be afraid to say "When I find out, I'll let you know" if you don't know the answers.

- **Why do you need that now?** – If you're not comfortable saying "I'd just like to be prepared," it's a good diversion to reference someone else: "My doctor/lawyer/spouse/partner thought it would be a good idea. You never know when you just may need them." This type of response may help you if you are not prepared to talk about another person's specific health situation.

- **How do you make those decisions?** – Many of these issues are volatile and can lead to serious arguments and hurt feelings. It's probably wise to not get into an involved discussion about how these decisions were made. Instead, tell them they should try talking it through with someone they trust; then writing things down; setting it aside and reviewing it at a later time.

- **What plans have been made?** – These details are highly personal and you need to decide how much you want to share. Share as much as you feel comfortable with. If the person is more of an acquaintance, you may want to generically mention the patient's medical treatment options.

- **Are you sure it's legal or it will be recognized as a legal document? Do you have to register or notarize it with anyone?** – Each state has its own completion and filing requirements. Check the document you are completing for information or talk to your lawyer, financial planner, doctor, or other planning professional to be sure.

- **Who has copies of that? Who will know or need to know about these requests?** – Generally, at least one other person – a spouse, a partner, or a close family/friend – should have a copy of Advance Directive documents, in addition to the person who completes the documents. If you're working with a planning professional (a financial advisor or an attorney), make sure she has a copy of them as well. Most states do not require that these be on file and available to the public.

Taking Care of Yourself

"She asked me if I did my own planning when we did it for Roger," says Karen, 52. "I didn't think about doing it right along with him. It hadn't been my first priority, but I can see now that it's a good idea to have mine done too."

Getting to know the patient and his wishes can be mentally and emotionally taxing for you. Remember that secret from Chapter 1 and balance your needs with the patient's needs. Here are some helpful hints to do that as you work with him on future planning:

- Think about and document your own wishes for future care, like Karen in the quote above. This way, you will be spending time together and completing both sets of directives, not just one.

- Try to be organized. It's easier to complete paperwork when you know where to locate it.

- Establish coping mechanisms for yourself, whether that's walking, gardening, or keeping a journal. Turn to them when you need them.

Lastly, don't underestimate the power of a good friend. If talking about these issues becomes tedious, get a friend involved to try another tactic with him. Don't forget to take a little break or celebrate with that friend when you make some progress.

Wrapping Up

You've done a lot of work! You've gotten to know the patient a little better after reviewing his personal and medical history. You've asked powerful questions about personal business and medical care. You've discussed sensitive subjects with the patient and you've formulated his desire for future treatment. By now, you're beginning to get a good understanding of how important a caregiver is: You're really involved in planning someone's life!

As you continue your journey, keep in mind:

- Even formal Advance Directive documents can be revised. If the patient changes his mind about treatment, you can update them and re-file them at any time.

- There are many ways to overcome objections or scrutiny from others. Use the suggestions from this chapter or script your own answers.

- Scheduling happy events is nearly as important as scheduling necessary ones. Laughter is, as the saying goes, the best medicine.

After reading this chapter, you're also probably realizing the value of other people and resources in the caregiving process. In the next chapter, we will address how to build a personalized CARE PLAN and CARE TEAM.

Chapter 3: Assembling Your Care Team and Care Plan

"We keep a group binder about our girlfriend," says Melinda, 38, whose friend Stephanie was diagnosed with colon cancer. "It has all her medical history in it. We take turns being with her, and whoever goes with her to the hospital or a doctor carries it and adds to it. If anyone has any medical questions about her, we know to look there first."

So far, you've been given a glimpse into caregiving responsibilities and the patient's wishes for future care. With that foundation, you will be able to figure out your next steps: what you and the patient are going to do and who's going to help you do it.

It's easy to feel lost without a plan. The goal of this chapter is to identify what medical and non-medical support you may need and to devise your personalized approach to care. Let's call these your CARE TEAM and CARE PLAN. We will create these in parallel as they are intertwined.

We will begin by first putting together the paperwork that you and the patient have received and continue with:

- Learning About Insurance Coverage

- Identifying Your Care Team

- Shaping Your Care Plan

- Taking Care of Yourself.

However simple or elaborate you want to make your Care Plan, you'll need some basic supplies: a folder or binder with pockets, some paper in a notebook or pad, and a pen or pencil. Bring those supplies and gather any patient-related paperwork you have: copies of medical records, ADVANCE DIRECTIVE DOCUMENTS, prescriptions, notes from doctor's visits, bills, insurance information, suggestions from friends, and so on. It's time to develop your plan of action.

Putting Together the Paperwork

"My sister was the one with the cancer, but I was the one that got the education," says Amy, 38. "Suddenly I was learning all these medical terms and facts, meeting all these medical people, and being shown all these procedures and machines. It got to the point that I thought if I did go to nursing school it would be very easy for me, because I had learned so much in the crash course of a cancer diagnosis."

The first step towards putting together a Care Plan is to review and understand the information that has been given to you or that you have discovered on your own. It may take some effort to put all of it together, especially when you have information coming from multiple sources.

In many places in this book, we will provide checklists. They are guidelines for you to use however they make sense to you. You may want to add other bullet points or omit some of the activity if it doesn't apply. Here's one to get you started in putting together the paperwork.

Checklist: Putting Together the Patient's Paperwork

☐	Put all of the patient's medical information in a folder or binder with pockets. This means literature, appointment cards, referrals, images, and other test results.
☐	Carry the folder with you for all interactions with the medical professionals. If you have one, use a tote bag to carry it back and forth.
☐	If the folder gets too heavy to carry, create a space at home where you can leave some of the non-critical paperwork behind.
☐	Whatever you and the patient decide about the treatment path, keep meticulous records in regards to appointment times and impacts to work (days off or sick time). Keep a calendar of cancer and non-cancer related events. It will give you both things to look forward to.
☐	When the bills start coming in, keep records of claims made, as well as claims paid. If you take careful notes of appointments and referrals, you can reference your notes and correct the information in the bills, if necessary.

When you're ready to go through it and organize it, do it at home. Do this when you can be alone and concentrate on it, even if that means just a few minutes at a time. Try following these steps:

Step 1: Lay out your paperwork out on a big workspace, like a desk or the floor.

Step 2: Divide paperwork into little sections. A big mass of paperwork can be overwhelming, so take a minute and separate it. For example, put all your notes or evaluations from doctor's visits, doctor referrals, and insurance information in one pile; lab test information in a second pile; x-rays and scans in another; and PATHOLOGY REPORTS from biopsies or surgeries in a third.

Step 3: Look at the notes and evaluations from specific doctors now and save the other piles for later – you'll have a chance to work on those a little later, while the patient is undergoing treatment.

Step 4: With your "Notes and Evaluations" pile, you'll probably have information about the DIAGNOSIS and what the doctor recommends. You'll need to figure out what each piece of paper means and if it requires action. Pick one up and decide if it is a general note that you took when the doctor was explaining something, a treatment plan or something to act on, a referral for a consultation with a specialist, or a request for a follow-up appointment.

Step 5: Then figure out what you need to do with it:

- Has it been discussed with the patient? If so, what did you two decide to do with it? If not, when is the right time to do so?

- If it is a request for another appointment, has it already been set up? Or do you want/need to make a phone call to do so?

- Do you want to get clarity on some terms or get a second opinion before doing any of that?

- Does it need to go to the recycle bin?

Step 6: Go through as much of the pile as you can. You may encounter a few stumbling blocks, like finding it hard to concentrate, or being unable to read a doctor's handwriting, or not understanding the information after you've read it. Take heart, you can usually call the doctor's office to help you decipher what's on the paper.

Step 7: Congratulate yourself, you did it! After you have reviewed the papers in this pile, you will be able to summarize what the medical professionals suggest that you and the patient should do. Then, you can start to uncover what eligibility and limitations the patient has through his insurance. Keep those referrals and recommendations together – but handy – in your folder. You will be developing the Care Plan using information on what the patient needs and what is covered by his insurance.

Learning About Insurance Coverage

"He says he has the best insurance in the world, but I know coverage changes," says Drew, 40, whose partner was diagnosed with prostate cancer. "What was covered yesterday may not be covered today."

Insurance coverage will guide your choice of physicians, specialists, facilities, and treatments. By knowing about the patient's coverage, you will understand if the insurance company is going to pay for part or all of the associated costs. In addition, you can avoid extra costs or confusion by working within the policy limits. The earlier you can gather and read insurance information, the better. You will need to find out what insurance the patient has (or does not have) and how that can be supplemented (if at all).

If the patient has insurance, get a copy of the policy, whether you are the policyholder covering the patient or not. In the United States, many kinds of insurance plans are available, but the four most common categories are: Indemnity, HMO, PPO and Self-Insurance. They vary on percentage paid toward care costs and which professionals they choose to work with (called "in-network"). See the Resource Directory in the back of this book for entities to contact with insurance questions.

When you have a copy of the policy, review it to become familiar with:

- Terms and coverage for current care, including doctors, specialists, facilities, hospital stays, transportation, treatments, equipment/prescriptions, or CLINICAL TRIALS

- How to file a claim and how to re-file a claim (if it is rejected)

- Coverage for future care as treatments begin and end

- Where you can go for patient advocacy

- Your main contact for referrals, pre-approvals, and billing.

Check to see if the recommendations for care are covered in the policy, as well as any restrictions on healthcare providers.

If the patient does not have insurance, he is not alone. However, it's important to remember that *cancer care is not free. If you and the patient decide to pursue a treatment without insurance coverage, you need to be prepared to pay for that treatment.* While the lack of insurance continues to be a nationwide problem, the patient does not have to fall into this category. Individual insurance policies are still available for purchase through large insurance agencies, even after a diagnosis has been made. Insurance premiums for those diagnosed with cancer are much higher than for healthy individuals, because the payout will likely be much higher. Still, it may benefit your financial situation to look into the possibilities of insurance for the patient before treatment begins.

There are also other programs that can help pay for this care. State and federal agencies (such as Medicare or Medicaid) may offer coverage or they may refer the patient to other agencies that do. Medicare provides for hospital/skilled nursing, but it does require a deductible, premium, and co-pay. Eighty percent of the outpatient expenses are generally covered; for the remaining 20%, Medicare can be supplemented with private insurance. Check with your Medicare representative about patient eligibility.

If the patient is uninsured and not eligible for these programs, you need to consider other options for care providers and treatment payment like paying for services out of pocket.

By putting together your paperwork and understanding your insurance situation, you've started on your Care Plan. Let's change gears for a moment and work on the Care Team. We'll get back to the Care Plan later in the chapter.

Identifying Your Care Team

> *"We chose that oncologist because we decided he would cut through all the B.S. and give us really great care," says Alexa, 37. "We also decided he probably wouldn't be the first guest invited to our cocktail party."*

After you have a handle on what the doctors recommend and you understand what the insurance will cover, your next step is to identify the other people – medical and non-medical – who can help you. No patient or caregiver needs to go through this alone.

When we talk about the patient's Care Team, we will include not just the medical professionals involved in a formal hospital or office setting, but also those friends and neighbors who will help you care for this patient. That means your sister-in-law who is in town for a couple of weeks or the person on your tennis team who brings over some macaroni and cheese for dinner are both a part of the Care Team. We'll talk more about building the patient's non-medical support network later in this chapter. First, let's talk about the patient's healthcare providers.

Professionals Involved in Cancer Care

One positive aspect of experiencing a common disease is that a variety of specialized professionals exist to facilitate patient care or be a support for you. The summary in the next section names the medical people that may be involved in the patient's care and the following table describes their responsibilities. When you have questions about the role of a medical professional, the table may provide answers for you. Keep in mind that medical doctors (MDs) have completed medical school, internships, and residency in their specialties and they are considered the most educated of all healthcare professionals. Doctors of Osteopathy (DOs) have completed equivalent medical training and may serve in the same capacities as MDs. Both are board certified.

The team involved in surgery can consist of:

- Surgeon or surgical oncologist, who prescribes it

- Assisting surgeon, on larger or complex operations

- Anesthesiologist or anesthetist, who administers anesthesia

- Scrub technician, who hands instruments and supplies to the surgeon

- Operating room nurse, who prepares the patient for surgery, collects appropriate equipment and material for the procedure, and documents procedure details

- Nurse practitioner (NP) or Physician Assistant (PA), who interfaces with the surgeon and addresses your questions

- Pre-anesthesia care unit nurse, who administers pre-operative treatments

- Post-anesthesia care unit/recovery room nurse, who monitors the patient immediately after procedure

- Support personnel.

The team involved in RADIATION THERAPY can consist of:

- Radiation oncologist, who prescribes it

- Radiation technologist or radiation physicist, who manages the equipment and works with other team members to precisely define the location and approach

- Dosimetrist, who calculates the amount, or dose, of radiation

- Radiation therapist, who guides the position of the patient for treatment and runs the equipment

- Radiation nurse, who coordinates treatment and addresses your questions

- Support personnel.

The team involved in CHEMOTHERAPY can consist of:

- Medical oncologist, who prescribes the dose and agents which will be used

- Nurse practitioner (NP) or Physician Assistant (PA), who interfaces with the oncologist and addresses your questions

- ONCOLOGY nurse (ONC), who coordinates treatment and addresses your questions

- Support personnel.

Explanation of Medical Personnel

Who Are These People and What Do They Do?

Title	Who They Are	What You Can Rely On Them For
Medical Oncologists/ Oncologists	Medical Doctors (MDs) or Doctors of Osteopathy (DOs) who practice the recognition and treatment of cancer (oncology). Oncology is a subspecialty of internal medicine. If they treat blood diseases, they are also called hematologists.	Medical oncologists look at the SYSTEMIC local affects of the disease. They also provide recommendations for treatment and monitor the patient's response to treatment. In complex cases, they may also recommend consultations with surgeons and/or radiation therapists.
Radiation Oncologists	MDs or DOs who primarily treat patients by use of radiation.	These oncologists regulate the type, location and dosage of radiation to kill or shrink CANCER CELLS.
Diagnostic Radiologists	MDs, DOs, or MD/PhDs trained to review imaging studies such as scans and X-rays.	These people help to stage the disease: show its location(s), growth pattern, and response to treatment. They may review initial studies or compare multiple studies.
Nuclear Medicine Physicians	These are specialty radiologists.	These MDs are trained to use radioactive substances for imaging.

Title	Who They Are	What You Can Rely On Them For
Surgical Oncologists/ Surgeons	A surgeon is trained to remove tissue and sew tissue together. A surgical oncologist has training in oncology beyond surgery, and specializes in removing cancer cells. Both can be MDs or DOs.	If the patient's cancer is considered RESECTIBLE, a surgeon will perform curative surgery by removing it from the body. A general surgeon may be called in to perform a non-cancer related surgery, such as removing the gall bladder or appendix.
Plastic Surgeons	These MDs work with skin, cartilage, fatty tissue and sometimes bone to reconstruct or change appearances or bodily function.	The patient may want to have cosmetic or RECONSTRUCTION surgery following a treatment (such as a MASTECTOMY or removal of a melanoma).
Nurse Practitioners, Physicians Assistants	Nurses who have advanced medical certifications or degrees, such as Masters in Nursing or Physician's Assistant License.	These professionals work with the patient on behalf of doctor. They are a wealth of information; can spend more time with you; are qualified to interpret lab reports; order tests and adjust medicine (all which are approved by a doctor).

Title	Who They Are	What You Can Rely On Them For
Oncology Nurses	Oncology nurses have additional training in the treatment of cancer.	There will likely be much communication with your doctor through your nurse, who acts as a relay about concerns and solutions. This nurse also administers chemotherapy in the medical oncologist's office.
Nurses, Nurse's Aides	Nurses have earned either BSNs (Bachelor of Science in Nursing) degrees, RNs (registered nurse) or PNs (practical nurse) licenses. Nurse's aides or CNAs (certified nursing assistants) may help with nursing duties as well.	The more education / specialty certifications the nurse has (college-educated and graduate work being among the highest), the more he or she will be able to facilitate care. If your hospital is a teaching hospital, you will likely encounter students of nursing. Nurses are in high demand and often stretched over multiple patients.
Psychologists, Psychiatrists, Social Workers	Psychiatrists are MDs or DOs; psychologists are PhDs and social workers are MSWs (Master of Social Work) or LSWs (Licensed Social Worker).	These professionals, like many of those listed above, must pass state boards to practice. Psychiatrists may dispense medicine, and all are trained in mental health. Some specialists address cancer-related problems.

Title	Who They Are	What You Can Rely On Them For
Pain Specialists	These MDs or DOs who evaluate the source and intensity of pain.	Not all facilities have pain specialists, but these helpful professionals recommend ways to stop or lessen pain, including non-prescription activity and prescription pain medicine.
Nutritionists/ Dieticians/ Naturopaths	The certification of these range from MS (Master of Science), RD (Registered Dietician) to Certified Nutrition Consultants. Most nutritionists and dieticians are state-licensed. However, only a few states currently have licensing requirements for naturopaths.	What the patient eats may affect treatment and recovery; likewise, treatments may affect eating patterns and nutritional needs. Nutritionists and dieticians work along side the oncologists to offer suggestions on managing changes or maintaining routines.
Pathologists	These MDs or DOs review tissue samples taken from the body during a BIOPSY or other surgery.	Most patients do not get to meet or choose the pathologist, but they are the professionals who actually make the DIAGNOSIS of cancer.

Title	Who They Are	What You Can Rely On Them For
Physical Therapists (PTs)/ Occupational Therapists (OTs)	PTs or OTs have years of training in kinesiology (human movement), anatomy, and physiology.	Therapists like these help to keep moving body parts functioning the way they should. They are especially important when the disease mandates a major alteration in musculoskeletal function.
Obstetricians/ Gynecologists, Urologists	Although you may not be having a baby or even planning one, these MDs or DOs are trained to safeguard your reproductive and sexual health through the disease and treatments.	Ask them for guidance on fertility and sexuality issues, especially with cancers of sex organs. They are also great sources of help for intimacy issues surrounding any type of cancer.
Endocrinologists	These MDs or DOs specialize in diagnosis and treatment of diseases related to the organs in involved in hormone production.	You may want their assistance if there is potential for damage to any hormone-producing entity or hormone-regulating entity.
Ears, Nose and Throat (ENT) Specialists	ENTs are other MDs or DOs that may be called to consult on issues affecting those areas.	An ENT can help with a number of ailments with the patient, from breathing to eating to hearing difficulties. Chemotherapy, surgery and radiation can impact these areas.

Title	Who They Are	What You Can Rely On Them For
Ambulance Personnel	These personnel are all medically trained usually as Emergency Medical Technicians (EMTs).	They have the very important jobs of preparing the patient for transport and driving to the hospital or other medical facility.
Medical Students, Residents, Fellows	Residents and Fellows are MDs or DOs at various points in formal training. Medical students are on their way to becoming independent practicing physicians.	If your hospital is a teaching hospital, you are likely to encounter these trainees, who will be an integral part of your care. If the patient has a rare form of cancer, he may be asked if more students can study him to learn.
Dentists	These Doctors of Dental Surgery (DDS) and Doctors of Dental Medicine (DMD) are equivalent to Surgeons and MDs or DOs (respectively) for the mouth and facial bones.	Especially helpful with head and neck cancers, dentists can help avoid or repair damage to teeth, cheeks, lips, tongue, and throat.
Geneticists	Geneticists are MDs or DOs specializing in heredity and gene make-up.	Researchers are actively investigating the genetic links and causes of cancers. Geneticists can also conduct genetic mapping, which can sometimes help predict the likelihood of different cancers.

Explanation of Support Personnel

Who Are These People and What Do They Do?

Title	Who They Are	What You Can Rely On Them For
Office Secretaries, Hospital Admission Personnel, Schedulers, and Discharge Planners	Don't underestimate how crucial these team members are. They are your gateways to medical care, and they can make this easy or difficult.	At doctor's orders, they may instruct the patient to come into the office for an appointment or go directly to the hospital for tests or admission. Be good to them and they'll likely return the favor.
Patient Advocates	Usually non-medical, the patient advocates talk to the medical team and insurance personnel about patient concerns	Patient advocates may offer different services, based on their specialty and training. Try asking them for help with referrals, insurance questions, and billing matters.
Spiritual Counselors	These can be rabbis, nuns, chaplains, priests, deacons, ministers, etc.	Many hospitals offer chaplains or other religious clergy on staff for spiritual guidance and counseling.
Volunteers	Coming from all walks of life, these people help out wherever needed. Many are cancer survivors.	You may be surprised at how many volunteers you run across: they can help to transport, entertain, listen and comfort the patient – easing all kinds of burdens on you.

When You Can Choose Your Primary Care Doctor or Specialist

You and the patient may not have much choice regarding the professionals who will be on your Care Team. If you are fortunate enough to be able to choose whom you will work with, you have many options. The insurance network will likely include the medical professionals to whom the diagnosing physician may refer the patient. It can be difficult to determine who will be right for the situation just by seeing the names of the professionals.

So, how do you find the right medical professional(s)? Try this:

First, think about the criteria you want in the professional. Then, make an appointment to meet those you have been referred to so that they may review the patient's condition.

The criteria you require in a medical professional may vary from person to person and even between caregiver and patient. The caregivers interviewed for this book were surveyed on character traits they most admired in physicians. They consistently came up with these five:

1. Trustworthy (qualifications, experience, certifications)

2. Compassionate (not patronizing, considerate of the whole person and his family)

3. Honest (doesn't withhold information)

4. Works within a reasonable timeline (lets you know when to rush or when you can take some time to think about it)

5. Accessible (returns calls, is available for appointments within reasonable period of time).

You will know what is comfortable for you. Just like any relationship, you must be able to trust them and to communicate with them.

What Do I Say? Checking Out a New Doctor or Specialist

When you're checking into credentials, you and the patient may also be curious to know if the doctor is well-versed in current research findings and if he will be supportive of any complementary efforts.

The best ways to find out about his credentials are to look up his background up on the internet and ask him. Use simple, direct questions like these:

- What training, board certification, and expertise does this doctor or specialist have?

- What does he do to stay current on research findings, medicines, or new techniques?

- What choices do we have?

- Why is this doctor the best for our specific situation?

To find out about his bedside manner, talk to other patients in the waiting room. Find out:

- What do other they say about him? Would they recommend him?

- How receptive is the doctor or specialist to complementary and alternative medicines?

- Will he suggest or approve other methods we are interested in?

There are many doctors and specialists that may be able to help you. When you have found one or two that seem to fit the bill, try them out. It's important to find the right one(s) for you.

A Few Words on Malpractice Information on the Internet

When you find malpractice information about a medical professional, read it with a critical eye. Sometimes, excellent doctors are named in a lawsuit even when they have fully conducted themselves within the STANDARD OF CARE. This is particularly true for doctors who deal with difficult cases or difficult patients.

In general, follow your instincts – if it doesn't feel right, ask more questions or find another doctor. You and the patient must feel that the doctor gives you appropriate respect, straight answers, and thorough explanations.

Second Opinions

> *"When I took my father to the second specialist, he had us do more tests," says Sharlene, 50. "After looking at those results, the doctor gave us a completely different response than our first doctor. I asked him right on the spot 'Why is this opposite of what we heard before?' He explained that the scans showed new growths as the cancer progressed, which is why we needed systemic treatment with chemotherapy instead of just surgery.*
>
> *He suggested sharing the new scans with our first doctor for our peace of mind, but not to dally. We did. Our first doctor agreed with the second diagnosis and we continued treatment with him. While both doctors welcomed second opinions, they also warned us that administration can cause delay in treatment and that it's critical not to put that on hold."*

Many people pursue second opinions on diagnosis and treatment options. Most doctors are not threatened by this; in fact, they may be willing to give you other names and phone numbers of colleagues that the patient could visit. Most people consider that getting a second (or even third) opinion is critical to identifying the right type of care. If you go for a second opinion, do not get it from another doctor from the same practice. Find a doctor in another practice who specializes in the patient's need.

Under ideal circumstances, Doctor Number 2 will arrive at the same diagnosis and recommendation as Doctor Number 1. If their findings are consistent, there are few questions about the next steps. However, there may be conflicting care recommendations, as Sharlene describes in the quote above. It can be disturbing when two trained professionals tell you two different things – you and the patient may be confused about which way to go.

A few things to keep in mind: What is everyone telling you to do? Why? Does it make sense to you and the patient? If one says one thing, and someone else says another, why is there disagreement? When this happens, if you have the opportunity to have the doctors compare their findings or to seek out a third opinion as a tie-breaker, do it. If you don't have the opportunity for the two doctors to discuss the case or for a third opinion, go with the professional and the type of treatment that gives you the most hope and that gives the patient the best chances for survival.

Cancer is a life-threatening illness and good healthcare professionals matter now. Build your Care Team with those who make you feel at ease. Do the research and check with other professionals to make sure they are the best for you and the patient.

When You Can Choose a Hospital or Other Care Facility

There are three general classifications of hospitals: teaching, non-teaching, and community. Teaching hospitals are associated with a medical school and are often at the forefront of medical discovery – they can usually grant you access to advanced technology. The staff members of a teaching hospital are equipped to tackle bigger, more complex problems than those in smaller hospitals. However, smaller hospitals may have affiliations with other healthcare facilities for specialty care not provided in-house.

Most people choose a care facility by its closeness to home, the doctor's ability to practice there, hospital specialties, and participation in the patient's insurance coverage. When you have the choice, look for a hospital where the procedures that the patient needs are done regularly with high success rates. Find a care facility with a good reputation or one you have a personal affiliation with.

Some web sites review hospitals and some groups evaluate health care systems and health plans as well. These evaluations are difficult and time-consuming to upgrade, which means that the material may be expensive but not current. Read this information with a critical eye as well.

After you have found the hospital, try to maintain consistency of care by staying with that hospital. However, if the patient is not comfortable at a particular hospital but is comfortable with his doctor, ask the doctor to refer you both to a different hospital, if possible.

A Few Words on Care Alternatives

Be cautious of facilities that offer "miracle cures" and "medical wonders." Facilities that are 'south of the border' may also have 'south of the border' regulation, licensing, and research to prove their methods work. While alternative and complementary medicines and care facilities have their place, don't be one of many that have been taken advantage of financially and emotionally. Do some investigation yourself before having the patient try what they offer.

Working with Medical Professionals

"Why can't his primary care doctor help him with his chemotherapy?" asked Arden, 66. "We trust him, after all these years."

Plainly and simply, you want the best care that the members of the patient's healthcare provider can provide. You want to optimize their education, experience, and access to technology and you want their maximum attention.

Unfortunately, so does everyone else.

So how do you make sure you accomplish that? You *don't* accomplish it by being argumentative or demanding. You *don't* accomplish it by crying or begging. You *do* accomplish it by optimizing each interaction. By being prepared. By building a rapport with them – a medical "partnership" – where both are upfront and honest.

Working well together begins with good interactions and conversations. Here are a few tips when talking to a doctor:

- It's up to you two to have up-to-date and accurate information for your doctor and other medical professionals. Have copies of all major reports with you at all times in case the doctor does not have them or if multiple doctors need to see the same reports.

- As one office suggests: "Talk so they will listen, listen as they are talking." That means when he's talking, take notes or use a tape recorder. Hear him, try to digest the information, and make sure that it makes sense. When you're talking, keep your questions defined, stay on track, and try to keep your emotions in check.

- If you or the patient is having difficulties in absorbing the information, ask if you can reschedule a time to finish the discussion. Older patients especially may experience memory loss or confusion, so if you need more time, ask for it.

- Ask your doctor to send copies of any written reports to the rest of the team so they are kept current.

- Remember that doctors are human and they have spouses, children, and other patients to attend to as well. They do not work 24 hours a day, seven days a week. Your doctor wants to know about you, but try to keep things pertinent to your healthcare concerns, unless he brings up other things.

When working with other medical professionals, remember:

- This is their environment – staff members know how things work on the inside and what shortcuts, if any, are available. Ask them how to best get things done.

- When possible, schedule appointments for early in the day. You won't have to agonize all day and there will be less chance that the doctor is behind or tired. Then you'll have the remainder of the day to relax or to take action.

- In your role as caregiver, you will also be the go-between with the medical professionals and the patient. Work with both of them on sharing information so that there are as few surprises as possible. Express fears to a team member in a listening role, such as a chaplain, social worker, nurse practitioner, or doctor. You will be able to determine the reality and probability of them and what you can do about them.

- Most importantly: *There should be one contact person (or two, at the most) that communicates with the doctor and staff.* It is not uncommon for other family members to temporarily relocate from other parts of the country to help the patient. Meeting with multiple family members on the same topic can be exponentially taxing on the staff, when the same information must be repeated multiple times. If you appoint one person as the key contact, it will make the time with the doctor more productive: he can spend more time on relaying new information instead of repeating the old.

Shaping Your Care Plan

"You've got to stay flexible. That's the key to caregiving,"
says Leanne, 55, whose husband has fought multiple cancers
and complications. "You learn something new every day,
encounter something different every day. So, you say this is
the plan today. This is the new plan. And you do that every
day, not bothering to think about yesterday's plan or how it
used to be."

Let's go back to your paperwork. You've sorted through the advice
from the medical professionals. You know what the patient's insurance
eligibility is and what treatment options you can pursue. You've
identified which specific medical professionals will likely be involved
in those various treatments and what facilities offer those treatments.
You and the patient have done a terrific job of managing the "behind
the scenes" activity.

Would you believe that you're almost done creating your Care Plan?
You are. When your Care Plan is "completed," you will use it to
make decisions on the patient's care and to delegate who will provide
assistance on both medical and non-medical issues.

The last few items in the plan complement what's happening on the
medical front. These are the actions that you and the patient will
do on the home front– with the help of a support network and with
the knowledge and approval of the medical members of your Care
Team.

Three critical components yet to be discussed are:

- Patient responsibilities

- Support network

- Community organizations and services.

Your Care Plan may have several other sections, based on the type
of illness and individual needs of the patient, but these are the core
parts. As mentioned earlier, your Care Plan can be as simple or as

ornate as you and the patient would like to make it. Many caregivers talk about the KISS principle: Keep It Short and Simple, because "The simpler it is, the more likely we will be to follow it." We'll talk about the patient responsibilities next.

Encouraging Patient Responsibilities

"Does she want to get up and take her medicine? No," *says Bradley, 76. "But she does want to get up to see the* *grandchildren."*

Yes, the patient is sick. Yes, she does need special attention and care. However, she also needs to do her part to increase the effectiveness of the medical care she receives. She can do this by committing to:

- Personal Research – becoming knowledgeable about the disease and its treatments. She can read books and medical publications, look online, ask support group attendees, and talk to health care professionals about the disease.

- Advance Directives – making sure these are up to date and accessible.

- Factual Conversation – preparing to talk about the illness, treatment, pain, and other symptoms in concrete, truthful terms. She cannot be shy or embarrassed about this if she wants the best help possible.

- Listen – asking for further explanation if she doesn't understand you or the Care Team.

- Instructions – realizing that "whatever you say" to the doctor or caregiver is sometimes appropriate, and arguing is rarely appropriate. If she wants to discuss an idea, concern or recommendation, she needs to boil it down to a few bullet points before bringing it up to the professionals.

- No Secret Maneuvers – alerting doctors or nurses if she chooses to investigate alternative or complementary methods of care (even vitamins) or if she refuses to follow directions, so that the medical professional can monitor the patient for interactions or changes.

As a caregiver, you can encourage her to fulfill these responsibilities by talking about them – even using this list as a conversation starter. Or, you may want to bring up her responsibilities as the circumstance strikes; for example, in the doctor's office, remind her of other symptoms she has shared with you that she is, for whatever reason, reluctant to share with the doctor. Of course, this sounds easier than it actually is, but keep trying. It will be helpful during the entire caregiving process.

What Do I Say? Interacting with the Patient

Whether you're at home, in an office, or at the hospital, your interactions with the patient can be challenging. It's easy to say be "normal," but that's difficult to do because this is not a normal situation. Here are some ideas that may help those interactions go more smoothly:

- Promises mean a great deal to the patient. Do what you say you're going to do, when you say you're going to do it. Disappointments are hard to handle.

- Try not to show expressions of pity, only concern.

- Be a good listener. That means listening with your whole self, not looking around the room or at your watch.

- Don't use your cell phone in the hospital. Period. Besides being rude to the patient, it may interrupt the electronics of some machines and is generally prohibited.

- Keep the conversation natural. It doesn't have to be intellectual; it could start with a joke or a smile.

Lastly, remember the power of silence. Sometimes just quietly being with the patient is support enough.

Building the Patient's Non-Medical Support Network

"I feel like saying, 'Here's a copy of my To Do list! Knock yourself out,'" says Bill, 46. "Since my brother got lymphoma, I'm overloaded with things to do for him and his family. But I can't forget my own responsibilities, too."

Frankly, it's time to call in the troops. Soon you'll start preparing with the patient for treatment and then managing the effects of the treatment. You need to start lining up who you can count on to fight this enemy. These are the people you will turn to – probably repeatedly – for assistance.

Choosing people to be soldiers with you can be difficult, because not everyone has the core strength or desire for the job. In addition, it may be hard for you to initially trust others with your feelings and patient care responsibilities, especially if you've been doing everything yourself. It might also be hard to trust others later in the process – if you've been burned because of some who have let you down.

When the news of the cancer diagnosis starts to spread, you'll probably have an immediate response from new recruits (like close friends or family members) who want to help.

You may have to draft others, including those who didn't initially want to be involved. Call in favors from the past. Did you take care of their dog when they went on vacation? Did you pick up their kids from school? Did you give money for a charitable cause? You helped them once, now it's your turn to be helped.

You may also have some volunteers who freely sign up to help. Volunteers have been known to unexpectedly surface, offering a variety of wonderful services like meals, child care, and transportation.

All of these people should be part of the Care Team. Don't turn anyone away. When you feel yourself resisting the help, *stop and think*: you need all the help you can get. Evaluate the possibility of them helping you instead of saying "no thanks, we've got this covered." Consider what they can do to help or where they would best fit.

The answer may lie in how well you know them. If they are relatives or friends, you may be able to gauge their behavior more readily than if they are strangers. Stranger or not, however, they may be well-meaning but ineffective. Or worse, they may be negative and bring more harm than good.

Remember that people are human; you may have to qualify the help a little:

- Are they dependable? Will they be there when they say they will?

- Where will their commitment end? Find out what their priorities are and where their life will get in the way of your requests.

- Are they the right person(s) for the job and will they address the patient's needs and privacy as you would?

When you reach your comfort level about a person, ask for a little assistance. Don't abuse your help either. If she says she can't help, it may be because she really is emotionally or physically unable to help. She may have time constraints. She may say "Yes" even though she really means "No" or "Not really." Evaluate the non-verbal communications (facial movements, eye contact, body posture, physical movement, or use of personal space) for clues regarding her level of interest.

She may not want to, but she may do it anyway, begrudgingly, just to avoid the discomfort of telling you "No." When you sense this, it's fair to ask "You don't really want to do this, do you?" to give her a way out. If she doesn't want to do it, she can say so, and you can find a substitute. Let her know that if she can't do it this time, you understand and you'd like to be able to ask for help another time.

Being able to depend on people is a terrific advantage and it should not be abused. You never know when you'll need help again, so be extra nice to those who help you.

A Few Words on Renegades Who Want to be Involved in the Care Plan

It's difficult enough to keep things on track when you know what direction you're headed. But when out of town guests, long lost family members, or other people appear who are suddenly interested in facilitating care – it can be a nightmare.

When family members argue (and too often, they do), each person probably thinks he or she is doing what is right. Siblings fight with other siblings; new spouses and step-children argue; or any two people who love the patient will go to war with each other instead of the illness. This can be terribly confusing or even detrimental to the Care Plan that has been crafted.

If they really have the patient's best interest in mind, evaluate what they're doing and saying. See how it fits in with the Care Plan. If it's helpful, fit it in. If it isn't, put it aside. You have been with the patient longer than they have and you will probably continue his care longer than those others are around. Your opinion holds more weight in the decision-making process and don't forget it.

What Do I Say? Talking to Others About the Patient's Progress

Other people in your circle may want to know what's happening with the patient. The next section offers suggestions on how to manage exchanges with them.

People will ask about the patient mostly because they care, they respect you, and they want to be courteous. So be prepared with a short, informative reply that reflects your appreciation for their interest.

Talk to the patient about what he would like you to say about the situation (unless the patient is unable to communicate). Find some phrases that are comfortable for you to explain the patient's status and what you're doing about it. A little bit of practice helps you deal with the questions when they come. Some typical questions and possible answers are given here. You may want to actually write out your answers, because this is new to you as well.

- **What's happening with the patient? How's she doing?** –Again, you can share details of the story as appropriate to the listener (that is, the closer the person, the more news you want to give out.) A simple "We're trying to get more information about the diagnosis and we'll let you know when we do" can work just great.

- **How did you find out?** – One- or two-sentence descriptions will suffice here. By keeping your answers short, you can limit the emotional toll that reliving the very beginning of this journey can have.

- **What do people do in that situation? What are you going to do next?** – If the person is caring and seems receptive to helping, tell her that you are finding out for yourself and ask her to research with you. This will keep those that don't want to help from asking in the future and enroll those that do want to help right away.

- **Is she terminal? Is she going to die?** – This question comes like a shot. Either way, the answer is emotional and be careful about how you respond. You may want to say "We don't know; the doctors are still determining that."

- **Maybe you should talk to Johnny. He does something in the medical field.** – A referral can be a wonderful thing, leading you to experts in the area of concern. However, sometime the referring person may unintentionally lead you towards someone that isn't a fit. Do some follow-up, on a limited basis, if you trust the source. If you find the referral applies, make a phone call or schedule an appointment.

- **How are you going to pay for this?** – If the person asking could help secure financial resources and you could use that help, schedule a time to talk about it. Prepare what you know the patient will need, the estimated costs, what you can pay for, and what you know you will need help paying. The more information you have at this time, the better. Otherwise, the old Southern practice of deflection can be the best response: "Let us worry about those little things."

Keep the patient's requests in mind and know that it's always OK to say: "I just can't talk about this right now, but I'll get back to you" or "I just don't know." Spend your energy on searching out helpful organizations and services instead.

Using Community Organizations and Services

"I don't know what I would have done if I lived anywhere else but here," said Erica, 60. "Everyone gathered around me as soon as they found out Ed was sick. I think every possible service offered a helping hand."

Because this disease is so widespread, national, regional, and local groups have been formed to manage the problems that surface. These organizations are excellent resources for both the patient and the caregiver. If you are searching to enhance your support network with experienced and local people, start by checking your phone book, newspaper, or the internet. Also look at the organizations listed in the Resource Directory in the back of the book.

While it doesn't include every organization, it includes general cancer organizations that can put you in touch with groups that are more specific to the patient's illness. After you are in touch with them, think about what you would like to get out of them: Emotional support? Information? Referrals? Treatment options? Encouragement and hope? Mental health or counseling resources? All of the above? Those services may be there for you – but you may have to do a little investigating or traveling to take advantage of them.

Additionally, hundreds of services have been established to help you solve cancer-related problems. The next few pages provide baseline information in the areas of: general services, hospital-based services, finances, insurance and legal concerns, transportation, and spirituality. Again, look for resources close to home or to the patient's care facility, so that you can more readily participate.

General Services

Depending on your location, the number of general services available to you and the patient can be either extensive or somewhat limited. Usually, organizations based in larger cities will reach out to smaller townships and suburbs, realizing the need exists there as well. Examples of these services are:

- Adult day care

- Boutiques and clothing stores, including those selling scarves or wigs

- Child care

- Handyperson services

- Home delivered meals, like Meals on Wheels

- Home health aides

- Homemaker or housekeeping services

- Hospital supply companies for first-aid supplies or equipment

- Lodging

- Specialty shops for prosthetics

- Service and support centers, like Civic Centers, Senior Centers, The Gathering Place, or The Wellness Center

Before you agree to take advantage of any support services, it is a good idea to do a little research. Find out about special programs, seminars, or workshops that are available. Most of these are offered at a nominal cost or free of charge and they can offer some very useful advice.

You'll also want to be sure that the organization or individual is reputable, that you can get the most from their offering, and that there will be no surprise fees after you have used the service. If you need a little help knowing what to say to the people in these organizations, see the next section.

What Do I Say? Questions For Support Services

When you are seeking help from organizations that you're not familiar with, try these sample questions:

- What services do you have for the patient or the caregiver that we could take advantage of?

- How does someone apply for these services? What are the eligibility requirements? And how many times would we be able to use you?

- What other kinds of patients use this service?

- What part of the services would I need to pay for? How much does that cost? If it's complementary, should I consider gratuity or tips?

- When can I anticipate this service? If something unforeseen happens, do you have a back-up?

- Do you work with any other organizations that may be valuable to us?

Remember that these services are often manned by volunteers – Again, many of them are cancer survivors who want to give something back to the community. So keep that in mind when dealing with them. They may be wonderful sources of inspiration to you and the patient, just when you need some!

Using Hospital-Based Services

Don't forget that hospitals, nursing homes, and other care facilities offer many services beyond medical treatment for the patient. These may include nutritional guidance, assorted training programs, conferences and other networking opportunities, counseling, support groups, cancer survivor networks, and survivorship celebrations. Many caregivers recommend attending survivor meetings and support groups for specific cancers as soon as possible so you can be with other people who may understand your situation.

Hospitals often host different types of support groups: Peer-led groups are facilitated by a cancer survivor; Professionally-led groups feature a medical or mental health professional; Spiritually-led groups are usually presented by a minister, priest, or rabbi who relies on experiences he has shared but not necessarily experienced first-hand. Most support groups are free. Try them out to see if they feel comfortable for you.

Finances

When someone has a health concern, especially a serious illness, it can bring two-part financial disaster. One part is income-earning impact, as the patient is too sick to work or he misses work because of treatments; the other part is the additional weight of medical expenses.

Sometimes it's difficult to ask for financial support. This is no time for pride, though – if you need it, ask for it, and keep asking for it as long as you need it.

Organizations have been formed to directly offer financial assistance (payment or partial payment) and to point the responsible party to reduced or free services on a variety of levels, such as:

- Federal: The Administration on Aging, Medicare or the Social Security Administration, and the Veterans Administration are available to assist with insurance, prescription, and general care needs. Call the local branch of these government departments to see if the patient qualifies for assistance.

- National: Several cancer-related groups have financial assistance programs for both patients and caregivers across the U.S. that demonstrate need. Look in the Resource Directory in the back of this book for cancer-related organizations.

- <u>Religious and Spiritual</u>: Houses of worship and service organizations have funds set aside and volunteers available to help members and their families who are fighting cancer. It's easy to overlook organizations with a religious or spiritual affiliation, but they are numerous and they can be influential, especially in smaller communities. Check your phone book for contact numbers.

- <u>State</u>: About half of the states have departments that are dedicated to financial assistance for low income or indigent patients and their caregivers. Look at the web site for your state government or search in the blue pages in the phone book for the names and numbers of those who can help.

- <u>Industry</u>: Many medical manufacturers and pharmaceutical companies and distributors provide financial programs for low-income families or indigent patients. See the Resource Directory for a few of these companies.

- <u>Corporate and Foundation</u>: Grants and other funds are earmarked for patients with specific cancers or for clinical trials and other research to cure specific cancers. Search the internet for options.

- <u>Financial Services</u>: Professionals including financial planners, social workers, and case administrators offer individual counseling, community programs, and financial planning workshops to counter existing pressures and to help manage upcoming expenses.

- <u>Debt Management</u>: Credit counselors can help with payment plans, debt settlement, loans, and other options to manage debt from both medical expenses and other sources that could not be paid while the patient was sick. Be wary though: some agencies are more credible than others. You may want to contact an organization to check the agency out before you ask for their help handling credit and payment issues.

- <u>Local</u>: Some utility companies will grant financial assistance or provide payment options when they are alerted of a serious illness in a household. In addition, some organizations will help with lodging needs for the patient, out of town family members, or others.

- <u>Individual</u>: Oncologists are sometimes given free samples from pharmaceutical companies through their representatives. Ask the oncologist if there are some samples of the patient's prescriptions.

Because of the great need for aid, there are often lines or waiting lists that you and the patient may be part of to utilize these services. Take heart: The key is to apply early and to apply to utilize as many as possible. Try to research and apply while you both have the energy – and before treatments begin for the patient – so he can fill out forms with you.

A Few Words on Viatical Companies

Viatical companies buy valid insurance policies for cash. Patients and caregivers sometimes sell insurance policies to help offset treatment costs. In the "life settlement" industry, patients may sell an existing life insurance policy for more than its "cash surrender value" but less than its "net death benefit." What this means is that the insurance company will pay money on the policy to the policyholder before the patient has died. The payout will be less than if the patient died, but more than if the policy were "surrendered," or cancelled, and the invested monies returned. Then, patients may have cash available when it is needed to pay expenses while they are living.

Insurance and Legal Assistance

A cancer diagnosis places a tremendous amount of dependency on a patient's (or his family/caregiver's) insurance policy. This policy influences decisions on care and providers, and affects the overall financial situation. Having a good relationship with your benefits administrator or insurance agent will help you in a number of ways, like:

- Answering questions on treatment and physician coverage

- Helping to file claims

- Following claim status.

However, if you need more help than that resource is able to provide, several others are around to help. Go to the claims director within your insurance company. Try the human resources personnel at work. Ask the social worker or patient advocate at the hospital. Talk to the patient advocate, social worker or office managers at the oncologist's office. Or, when an issue is particularly serious, contact your State Insurance Commissioner's office. Don't stop until the issue is resolved. It may not be resolved to your satisfaction, but at least you gave it your best shot.

Keep in mind that inexpensive (or even free!) legal resources exist to help fight civil (not criminal) matters related to a cancer diagnosis or treatment. Check your phone book or the internet for organizations like the Cancer Legal Initiative or the Breast Cancer Legal Initiative.

Transportation

The patient may be too weak or too sick to take himself to treatment or check-ups. When you have other responsibilities, you may need some assistance with – or reprieve from – the transportation duties. In addition to asking friends or family members for help, look into these other options:

- Volunteer transport organizations, shuttle services between care facilities, vans from community centers to hospitals, free shuttle services to grocery stores and pharmacies

- Carpooling with other patients

- Low-cost or free transportation for elderly or disabled

- Private transport in private cars or taxis

- Round-trip rail tickets to cancer events or facilities

- Plane fare or free flights through private providers.

Another handy tip: Shop around for rates on taxis or airfare. Ask for a "book of tickets" or a discount rate if you know you will need to purchase round trips or multiple trips to certain facilities in the immediate future.

Spirituality

Finding a spiritual resource has anchored and strengthened a number of caregivers who were interviewed for this book. Patients and caregivers may be reluctant to talk about their respective faiths, as spiritual needs can be extremely personal. On the flip side, others may want to be extremely vocal about their faith. Fortunately, members of clergy are usually accessible in a care facility if you do want to talk or vent in confidence – and they rarely charge for listening. You may also be interested in spiritual renewal programs offered through individual places of worship and other support centers.

Starting to Use Your Care Plan

> *"What about caregiving is easy?" says Moya, 61. "Delegation."*

You've collected lots of wonderful information for your Care Plan binder, including names, phone numbers, and services. So how do you know when to stop creating and start using it? The answer is you've already started using it to make good decisions on care. You will use it more as you tend to the patient during and after treatment, as you'll see in later chapters. It may be difficult to stay on top of all the current service offerings as new ones continue to surface. You'll quickly learn what works for you and the patient and you can always modify your Care Plan.

Taking Care Of Yourself

"I'd lost about 30 pounds taking care of my husband," says Marilyn, 56. "It wasn't until after he'd passed that people noticed."

Here you are, creating a Care Plan and assembling the Care Team for the patient. You may be juggling work and family concerns as well – do you even have time to understand and manage how you feel? Self-care is often last on caregivers' lists, with the patients' needs taking the top spot. So much focus is placed on the patients that the caregivers become part of the background and their needs go unaddressed.

As they listen to the patients' prognoses, caregivers often begin to consider their own mortality. Natural fears about their own futures start to sink in, such as how they personally will be cared for, especially if the patient is the financial provider in the house; how their children will be cared for; how the disease will affect their own careers; and how the disease will affect other family members.

In addition, the feeling of guilt may be incredibly powerful. As a primary caregiver, you may be feeling guilty for being able to maintain the "normal" life you had or guilty about wanting to protect it from the impacts of the illness. You may even feel guilty for being in good health yourself. That's perfectly natural.

This situation is a lot to deal with – don't underestimate it. Because these issues can be mentally draining, you may not be as effective as you would normally be. It may be difficult to concentrate on the patient until you address your own thoughts and fears. Some other recommendations from fellow caregivers are:

- **Don't feel helpless**. Ask and keep asking for help. There is no shame in wanting or needing to take a break; it may be good for the patient as well.

- **Keep a gratitude journal to remember the good things.** Although it may be hard to come up with some entries, going back through the journal will help you deal with the tougher times, and you can create an heirloom with loving memories.

- **Do something to mentally remove yourself from the situation:** Sleep in, go for a walk, meditate or pray, sit in a rocking chair, be with children, play in the snow, put up decorations for holidays or special events.

- **Plan a vacation.** It doesn't mean you need to take it right away, and you can make it as exotic as you want. You may plan things, even an entire journey, that you never even take.

- **Don't 'suck it up.'** Find a person you can complain to or commiserate with and vent. If you need to let it all out privately, hold it in until you get to a "safe" place, like your car or the parking lot. Be safe, though: walking or driving with tears streaming down your face can impair your vision, and you don't want to be in the hospital, too.

If you seek more help with dealing with issues, there are many venues you can pursue, like private counseling, books, or peer groups. You may have to do a little research to find peer groups specific to your disease of interest and determine what the main focus of the group is (information, sharing, or advocacy). The key is to "try before you buy." Consider sitting in the back of the room, or listening outside the session. Don't be afraid to leave a session or group if it doesn't feel right.

With most groups, you can control your time and involvement to ensure you enjoy going and it does not become another "task" for you to complete.

What Do I Say? Questions for a Support Group

Try asking another attendee some of these questions to get you started:

- "How often do they have these meetings and how often do you come to them?"

- "Do you have any recommendations on financial aid or short-term counseling at a reasonable rate?"

- "What is happening in your situation?" "Do you feel any of these things I am feeling?"

- "Do you really give people an honest response when they ask you 'What can I do to help?' and how do you know if they really mean it?"

Other resources "at your fingertips" are there as well: try calling a friend, talking to an anonymous contact at a cancer hotline, or writing down your concerns. Problems may not seem so large when you talk or write them out.

Wrapping Up

You're on the right track! You've encouraged the patient to follow through with his responsibilities. You've identified a Care Team of talented medical professionals and non-medical people you can count on. You've gone through dozens of possibilities for assistance in your Care Plan. What a terrific job you're doing.

Keep going. Trust your instincts that you've covered the *big* bases. Keep lists of services and directories that you don't need right now for times when you may need them in the future. Remember that you may need to update or enhance your Care Plan as you research treatment options together. The next chapter guides you through collecting and analyzing that research.

Chapter 4: Researching Treatment Options with the Patient

"I'm no dummy, yet I'm having trouble understanding what all these words mean," says Patricia, 47, whose husband has multiple myeloma. "It's like you have to know the code words to get in to a secret society or something."

When you're making some decisions about treatment for a serious illness, you'll find yourself facing unfamiliar terms and explanations. The vocabulary that is spoken in a healthcare setting can be very complex and learning it can be very difficult.

The goal of this chapter is to give you a base understanding of traditional and non-traditional treatment options. This way, you'll be more comfortable when you and the patient are choosing what's right for your situation. We will discuss:

- Traditional Medical Treatments

- CLINICAL TRIALS

- Alternative and Complementary Approaches

- The Choice of Non-Treatment

- Taking Care of Yourself.

As you read this chapter, you'll notice that it contains a lot of medical information. Because of that, it may sound somewhat scientific. Read slowly and repeat if you need to. Words that may need more explanation appear in SMALL CAPS and can be found in the Glossary.

For the traditional therapies of SURGERY, RADIATION, and CHEMOTHERAPY, the sections pertaining to surgery are presented first; sections pertaining to radiation are second; and sections pertaining to chemotherapy are presented third. Some sections may not apply to you, so feel free to skip over them.

Treatment choice is highly personal. Some patients want to just follow "doctor's orders." Others want to actively participate in their own care, pursuing all options available. A few patients just want to the disease to follow on its normal course without treatment. If this is the case, please read the section later in this chapter entitled *"The Choice of Non-Treatment."*

It's important that the patient has time to evaluate all of the treatment options and that he doesn't feel pushed into a decision. Unless the patient has granted you Healthcare Power of Attorney, it is his choice to have treatment or not. He has the right to choose between the available options.

You can lend support by gathering information and helping him explore his objections or concerns, which we'll cover in this chapter. There are some complex areas ahead. Good luck. You'll be just fine.

Learning About Treatment Options

By now, you've probably sorted through various recommendations from the medical professionals. You also know about your insurance eligibility. You've narrowed down what treatment options you can pursue, and you've identified which specific medical professionals would likely be involved in those various treatments.

Your next step: Research. Cancer patients typically have quite a few options. The goal is to find credible information on the options that make sense for the patient. Put your investigative energy into finding therapies that could be right for your situation. Don't spend time researching one therapy if the oncologist is recommending another. Try these ideas:

- Review the brochures about illnesses and treatment options that are displayed in the oncologist's office.

- Search hospitals, clinics, and other healthcare facilities for reference rooms or lending libraries. These areas often have treatment summaries or worksheets for patients and caregivers.

- If you have internet access, go to web sites with treatment information. Start with a search engine and type in the specific treatment type or specific cancer type.

You and the patient can research together or separately. The patient may feel less worried and more in control when he is actively collecting information. He also may retain more knowledge if he is researching at his own pace, in ways that he can understand.

When it's time to compare notes, patients usually want to discuss the types of treatments available as well as the pros and cons of each. However, if the patient you're caring for doesn't want to research or talk about it, that's OK too. Consider having some summary information within his reach, just in case he wants to do a little reading. The next few sections may fit that purpose nicely, as we overview the common types of treatment. Let's get started.

Understanding Traditional Medical Treatments

In the United States, doctors are licensed to practice medicine within certain boundaries, called the "STANDARD OF CARE." This means that for any abnormal physical condition or malady that requires medical care, there is a specific way or ways that it should be treated. These are accepted methods because they cause the least harm and bring the greatest benefit to the patient. Standards of care are continually reviewed and tested as new methods, devices, and drugs are created.

The medical treatments comprising the standard of care for cancer patients include surgery, radiation and chemotherapy. These are called traditional treatments. You may hear medical professionals refer to them as MODALITIES. The objectives of traditional treatments are to remove growths, to keep TUMOR growth under control, or to prevent

RECURRENCE. Traditional treatments may be given by themselves or in combination, depending on the location and the stage of the cancer.

Many other methods of treatment exist, such as hormone therapy, IMMUNOTHERAPY, antibody therapy, and tumor biology. These are at various stages of acceptance into standard of care; and, depending on the cancer type and location, they may be viable options. We will also discuss them briefly.

Usually, oncologists lead the patient's other medical professionals and guide the patient on treatment choices. When making recommendations to the patient, the oncologists will review a variety of information. This includes the type and stage of the cancer, the general health and age of the patient, the patient's MEDICAL HISTORY, various quality of life issues, and possible SIDE EFFECTS of treatments. Further, they may evaluate response rate of a treatment, SURVIVAL RATES, possibility of major complications, and economic burden. Through training and experience, most oncologists can readily present more than one treatment option for most disease types. However, they may only present the best option in their medical opinions.

Prescribing care for cancer patients is complex, and it's understandable that the patient would have some confusion, worry, or nervousness about making treatment choices. Before pursuing any treatment, be sure to arm yourselves with as much information as possible. Read on for some items to discuss with the medical professionals of the patient's CARE TEAM.

What Do I Say? Being an Effective Advocate for the Patient

When you're going through treatment recommendations with a medical professional, talk about these subjects. Before committing to any procedure, be sure you understand the:

- procedure, risks and complications

- usual recovery time

- survival results and statistics

- description of any changes to expect after the procedure, both short- and long-term

- experience of the medical professional

- possible limitations on future treatment options

- cost of the procedure that you or the patient will be responsible for paying

- next steps after the treatment has been completed

- options if the treatments don't seem to be working.

To complement what you've learned from the medical professional, read the summaries about each treatment type. We've included *Benefits* and *Items to Consider* with each. Not all options are included, so check with the patient's oncologist for upcoming research, technology, or medicines that may benefit the patient.

Surgery

"My friend, who plays in a band, found a lump on his lip," said Shana, 32. *"The tumor grew to the whole side of his face, and he had to have it removed. They had originally told him the cancer was terminal, but it wasn't. They were able to operate on it. He had the cheek area and part of his gum and lip taken out. Then he had plastic surgery to repair everything and he's OK. He's just 38, with a wife and two kids."*

Many consider surgery to be the most successful weapon in the fight against some cancers. Surgery may be performed to detect cancer (BIOPSY), remove a tumor (RESECTION), reduce the size of a tumor (DEBULKING) or rebuild lost TISSUE (RECONSTRUCTION). Surgery is a LOCALIZED treatment, that is, it is intended for one place, or location, in the body. Surgeries are frequently recommended for breast, colorectal, prostate, lung, and skin cancers.

Types of Surgeries

Generally, there are two types of cancer surgery: OPEN SURGERY and MINIMALLY-INVASIVE surgery. In open surgery, a body cavity is opened with an incision. The surgeon and assistant look directly into the operative area or "field." Open surgeries are named for their location and activity. Those that end in –otomy mean "cutting into" and those that end in –ectomy mean "removal of." Examples of this are thorocotomy (cutting into the chest for lung cancer) and lobectomy (removal of a lobe for liver or lung cancer).

In minimally-invasive surgery, the surgeon makes several smaller incisions instead of one large incision. Through these incisions, small tubes (called ports) are inserted into the body cavity. Cameras and other instruments are brought into the operative field through these ports. Then, the surgeon can view the operative field and operate with the small instruments, without totally opening the body cavity. This usually results in decreased surgical trauma and shorter recovery time.

Benefits of Having Surgery

- Surgery can successfully remove or treat a wide variety of cancers. This includes using surgery to place devices that allow access to the different systems or cavities in the patient.

- The results are almost immediate. When the operation is finished and the PATHOLOGY REPORT is read, the patient and caregiver can know the findings.

- Surgery may also provide relief from a complication of the cancer, such as an obstruction or bleeding.

Items to Consider

- There is a possibility of complications with any surgery. These include infection, loss of blood, adverse effects of anesthesia, or scarring where the surgery took place, known as the INCISION SITE. When the procedure or side effects that surface later have greater risk than the cancer itself, other therapies may be recommended.

- To improve results, surgery may be followed by chemotherapy or radiation or both.

- Removal of body tissue can cause change in organ function, resulting in challenges with breathing, movement, digestion, sexual activity or fertility if the procedure targets an organ or gland connected to the reproductive process.

- Cancer does not spread (METASTASIZE) when it is exposed to the air. There is a common belief that as a result of the operation, it will spread throughout the body. Cancer metastasizes in other ways, usually through the patient's LYMPHATIC SYSTEM or circulatory system.

- Patients sometimes experience a psychological adjustment after a surgery, even if the changes are not visible, like "I'm a different person because one of my breasts has been operated on." It may be helpful to talk about the procedure with a social worker or counselor to work through the issues.

This information can assist you in setting your expectations for the success of the surgery. In Chapter 6, a sample surgical experience is outlined. You may want to read it with the patient as well.

Radiation Therapy

"With my wife's breast cancer, we made the serious decision to have radiation," said Tom, 68. "After her treatment, my grandson asked my wife if she was 'radioactive' now. He said he saw it on cartoons. It gave us a much-needed chance to laugh. We could tell he was slightly disappointed that she wasn't that kind of superhero."

Shortly after Roentgen's discovery of x-rays in the 1890's, researchers began to evaluate potential use of it in treating cancer. They found that radioactivity in the form of x-rays or gamma rays can be beneficial in treating cancer. Over time, studies showed that high-energy x-rays damaged CANCER CELLS, resulting in tumor cell death (albeit with side effects). With decades of research behind it, radiation has been successful in treating hundreds of thousands of patients with cancer. It is now regarded, along with surgery and chemotherapy, as one of three standard treatments for cancer.

RADIATION THERAPY (also called Radiotherapy) is used to:

- destroy cancerous cells

- reduce the risks of recurrence or METASTASIS

- reduce the size of the tumor or to kill remaining cancer cells after surgery or chemotherapy

- reduce symptoms such as pain or pressure brought on by the growth of the cancer cells, even when the cancer is considered incurable.

The goal of radiation therapy is to precisely target the radiation to the cancer cells while avoiding damage to other healthy organs and tissues. This is a very complex procedure. The cancer tumor may be small or in a hard-to-reach location. It may also be surrounded by vital organs like the brain, lungs, or heart. It is critical to decide exactly how the therapy will be administered for maximum benefit to the patient.

This therapy is often used with surgery. When used before surgery, radiation helps to shrink the tumor or inhibit new growth. During surgery, it helps to kill active cells. After surgery, it helps to stop growth in cancer cells that remain.

Radiation therapy is usually given as a localized treatment, like surgery. It is given in targeted doses to a specific site, called the "FIELD OF RADIATION" or "radiation port." This site varies with the location and complexity of the cancer.

Less commonly, radioactive compounds can be given SYSTEMICALLY, or throughout the body. That means that a patient may receive it INTRAVENOUSLY (IV), by mouth (as a pill) or by injection into a body cavity or the bloodstream. This method is prescribed for certain cancers such as thyroid cancers and as palliative therapy (comfort care) for patients with certain cancers (such as breast, lung, or prostate) metastasizing to the bones. In addition, radiation can be given by an external machine to the patient's entire body in certain instances with chemotherapy for stem cell or bone marrow transplants.

Types of Radiation

Two major categories of radiation are EXTERNAL BEAM and Internal Therapy (also called IMPLANT or Brachytherapy). Doctors specially trained in radiation and ONCOLOGY, Radiation Oncologists, will guide the patient in radiation decisions.

External Beam

External Beam radiation is administered from outside the patient's body. A specific machine generates radiation beams (rays) that are targeted to a specific body site in the patient. These machines incorporate computers for improved accuracy in directing the beams to hit the cancerous area. The beams kill some cells and prohibit the division of other cells. This procedure is usually painless to the patient.

Radiation is routinely administered five days a week, for a period of several weeks or more. The reason for this is to provide an opportunity for healthy tissue to recover from radiation damage. The patient can normally return home after each treatment. Caregivers are not permitted in the room as the patient receives radiation to avoid radiation exposure. In fact, for certain types of radiation, the radiation oncologist will recommend that caregivers provide some distance between themselves and the patient following treatment.

Internal Therapy

Internal Therapy (or Brachytherapy) can be thought of as a combination of surgery and radiation. In this procedure, radiation sources are placed inside the patient's body. These come in the form of capsules, pellets, or thin wires, and time-release the radiation at the center of the cancer. Two types of this treatment are intracavity radiation and interstitial radiation. Radiation sources may be introduced into a patient so they are inside a body cavity closest to the tumor (called intracavity radiation) or into the tumor itself (called interstitial radiation). Intracavity radiation is typically used in gynecologic tumors, and interstitial radiation is typically used in prostate cancers and sarcomas.

Because the placement and removal of these sources are considered surgeries, other people will not be permitted in the operating room. Even as the caregiver, you may not be allowed to be near the patient while the radiation sources are in place, as they could be potentially harmful to you. Talk to the radiation oncologist about safely interacting with the patient.

Benefits of Using Radiation

- Treatment time is fast (usually last less than one hour) and painless.

- Radiation can be valuable in reducing bone pain, with usual response rates between 80-85%.

99

Items to Consider

- Radiation can damage some healthy cells as it destroys cancerous cells. Tissue damage varies from organ to organ and depends on the area radiated as well as the dose. A higher dose may cause greater damage.

- RADIOPROTECTORS exist to block radiation from hitting healthy cells. These are commonly used for gynecologic and lung cancers. There may also be special precautions to protect the patient's skin during or after treatment. Talk to the radiation oncologist on your Care Team about this.

- Some side effects are immediate, such as changes to the skin around the site (blistering, darkening, swelling, inflammation). Other possible side effects include:

  o Fatigue

  o Voice impairment, loss of salivary function, mouth sores

  o LYMPHEDEMA (following breast cancer treatment)

  o Decrease in mental sharpness and clarity (following whole brain irradiation)

  o Loss of appetite, nausea, vomiting and bloating

  o Diarrhea, incontinence, and cramping

  o Intestinal obstruction (also called small bowel obstruction)

  o Cough

  o Nerve/spinal cord damage (less than 1%)

  o Second cancers (less than 1%).

- Patient will not be allowed to use certain soaps, deodorants, cosmetics, sunscreens, powders, lotions, or perfumes before radiation. These can contain certain chemical or metallic ingredients that may interfere with the radiation beams. Other toiletries that have drying ingredients, such as alcohol, may not be recommended because they increase the drying effect already present on the patient's skin with the radiation.

- Some effects may show up later – months or even years after treatment. The lungs, liver, eyes, stomach, bladder, and central nervous system are key areas to watch for damage.

Because the techniques used to give radiation are so varied, there are varied side effects. Generally, side effects are limited to tissues encompassed by or adjacent to the radiation field. You should have an idea of what will take place in your situation so you know what to what to expect after it is finished. This is important for both single dose and multiple dose treatments. Discuss the exact procedure with the healthcare team and read the section about typical radiation appointments later in Chapter 6. It will give you and the patient preparation ideas as well.

Chemotherapy

"When my daughter Erica started losing her hair, I cut mine," says Carol, 50. "When she lost it all, I shaved mine right along side her. It was liberating somehow. She had all kinds of fun hats and scarves to wear, and was a whiz with make-up – she managed to look good and find joy in the middle of this experience."

Some cancers can be cured by chemotherapy alone. Chemotherapy has been used for decades to treat cancer (in its many forms) by distributing chemicals throughout the body via the bloodstream. Chemotherapy is usually given as a systemic treatment; that is, it affects the whole body and its many systems. By not focusing on a single location, chemotherapy can:

- simultaneously destroy cancer cells in multiple sites through the patient's body

- stop cancer from spreading or decrease the risk of recurrence or of metastasis

- reduce or relieve symptoms caused by cancer, such as pain or pressure

- shrink tumors to supplement surgery or radiation.

Chemotherapy comes with its own vocabulary. With the different types of administration (localized or systemic), there are different types of chemotherapy REGIMENS. A regimen identifies what chemicals, or agents, will be used. Examples of regimens are single agent chemo, combination chemo, and chemo as part of a MULTIMODALITY approach. Single agent uses one cancer-fighting agent. Combination chemo uses more than one cancer-fighting agent. Multimodality approach means that other modalities, such as surgery or radiation, will be used with the chemotherapy to fight the disease.

Oncologists will recommend the regimen that is FIRST LINE THERAPY. This therapy is accepted as the most successful treatment PROTOCOL per disease type. This is the best treatment option that an oncologist can present. The first line of treatment is enough to safely treat most patients. However, the oncologist may prescribe a second line, third line, or more if needed. These lines may include another anticancer drug, drug combination, or MODALITY.

Chemotherapy is generally given in doses through CYCLES. Different treatment cycles and doses offer oncologists the ability to precisely tailor chemotherapy for a variety of diseases and patients. How the drug is given and how the patient responds to the treatment determine the length of these cycles. These recommendations constitute a protocol.

Chemotherapy is usually given by injection or IV. Hickman catheters, PORTACATHS, central lines and PICC lines are all examples of IV lines. Chemotherapy is also available in pill form, like other prescriptions, to treat some forms of cancer. The oncologist will guide the patient in determining the best way to receive the medicine.

Benefits of Using Chemotherapy

- With chemotherapy as a primary treatment, many people with cancer are living longer, and REMISSION or cure rates are higher.

- Chemotherapy generally lowers the possibility of recurrence.

- Cells that have spread from the original cancer site can be killed with chemo before they manifest into metastasis at another site of the body.

Items to Consider

- Side effects are a major concern to many cancer patients, such as:

  o Temporary hair loss. A number of chemotherapy drugs impact rapidly growing cells, including those in the skin, nail beds and hair follicles. This results in slow healing in the skin, slow growing of the nails, and hair loss.

  o Eating problems, including loss of appetite, nausea, and vomiting

  o Mouth sores and throat sores

  o Cognitive and memory changes, often called "CHEMO BRAIN"

- Chemotherapy has been shown to affect fertility in patients, up to and including permanent infertility. If the patient is within child-rearing years and interested in the possibility of having (more) children, ask the patient's doctor to take fertility preservation measures.

- There are many medicines and solutions available to counter the delayed complications of chemotherapy.

To set expectations about what will happen during a chemotherapy appointment, a "sample" chemotherapy experience is outlined in Chapter 6. You may want to read it with the patient to prepare for the experience.

Bone Marrow Transplants and Stem Cell Transplants

Patients receive bone marrow transplants (BMT) or stem cell transplants (SCT) to replace or restore healthy marrow that was destroyed by another treatment such as radiation or chemotherapy. Bone marrow is the substance inside bones that produces stem cells. Stem cells are naturally present in bone marrow and the blood. They mature into red blood cells, white blood cells, or platelets.

Benefits of Having BMT or SCT

- Higher than usual doses of chemotherapy can be to be given to the patient to improve the response rate and survival if his marrow is reconstituted.

- Filtering the blood and marrow, which is part of BMT and SCT, allows cancerous cells to be removed.

Items to Consider

- The patient's body may reject the transplanted marrow cells.

- Harvesting marrow or stem cells can be painful.

- The transplanted marrow (graft) may attack the patient's body (host) as if it were foreign (GRAFT VS. HOST DISEASE).

Immunotherapy, Tumor Biology, and Antibody Therapy

A substantial amount of research has been conducted in the areas of immunotherapy, tumor biology, and antibody therapy. Scientists continue to study ways to change cancer cells or the body's way of fighting them, including:

- understanding how mechanisms in cancer cells work

- altering traditional therapies like chemotherapy to not attack healthy cells and to more effectively attack cancerous cells

- encouraging cancer cells to act more "normal" with controlled dividing and dying

- increasing the ability of the patient's own immune system to fight cancer.

Other biological agents are being investigated to combat specific abnormalities that have not been identified in normal cells.

Developments with these and other upcoming targeted therapies will be tracked for inclusion in later editions of this book.

Benefits of Using Immunotherapy, Tumor Biology, or Antibody Therapy

- Immunotherapy and antibody therapy may potentially be less harmful than other forms of treatment.

- The patient may experience a higher degree of success as the first line of treatment, so that additional treatments may not be needed.

- Used with chemotherapy, these treatments can produce a higher response rate.

Items to Consider

- The results of these studies are mixed. Some immunotherapy has been shown to be effective and is incorporated into usual treatments. Some has not.

- Because these therapies may be specialized, they can be very expensive and not usually covered by insurance.

Hormone Therapy

Hormones control certain activity in the body and can feed certain types of tumor cells. Hormone therapy (also called endocrine therapy) can either block or stimulate production of hormones. It can also block the action of the hormones on tumor cells. When the receptors are *stimulated*, the hormones are distributed in the body and activity within the cells begins. When they're *blocked*, the hormones are not received. Then, the activity that they would normally have started does not begin.

Because of its activity in the body, this therapy can be thought of as "anti-hormonal therapy." That is, medicines are introduced into the patient to block the receptors for estrogen and testosterone for treatment of breast, uterine, and prostate cancers.

For example, some substances may be administered to block the activity of estrogen, thereby limiting the growth of the breast cancer cells that depend on estrogen for survival. The estrogen is still produced, but the activity it controls will not be started.

Other hormone therapies work differently, such as an "AROMATASE INHIBITOR." These medicines block the production of a hormone. An example of use of this is when testosterone production is blocked to combat growth of prostate cancer cells that depend on testosterone for survival. Like antibody therapy and immunotherapy, hormone therapy continues to be studied.

Hormone therapy is frequently used in tandem with chemotherapy or radiation. It should not be confused with Hormone Replacement Therapy. Hormone Replacement Therapy (HRT) has been prescribed to women in menopausal years. In HRT, estrogen is paired with progestin to replace hormones that are no longer produced in the body.

Benefits of Using Hormone Therapy

- Hormone therapy capitalizes on the body's natural mechanisms to protect, fight, and heal.

- Used correctly, hormone therapy can be used pre-treatment to protect fertility.

- Hormone therapy usually has fewer side effects and is better tolerated by patients.

- This therapy can usually be taken by mouth in pill form.

Items to Consider

- Side effects in men include a decrease in sexual desire, enlarged breasts, hot flashes, impotence, incontinence, and osteoporosis.

- Side effects in women include fatigue, hot flashes, mood swings, nausea, osteoporosis, and weight gain.

Multimodal Therapies

You've read summaries of different types of treatments. A variety of combinations may be used to fight a particular cancer. When treatments are used together, it is called MULTIMODAL THERAPY. The goal of multimodal therapy is to increase the effectiveness of individual treatments and help counter side effects.

The upcoming sections talk about how these individual treatments became proven treatments in a process called Clinical Trials.

Considering Clinical Trials

Just as the name implies, clinical trials are research programs conducted with patients in a clinical (or medical) setting. This research is how doctors and other medical professionals are able to determine better ways to detect cancer, stop cancer growth and treat cancer patients.

Clinical trials may involve a new drug or series of drugs, new devices, or new methods for giving an existing treatment. They may even test a combination of these. It is through clinical trials that any procedure, tool or pharmaceutical becomes a standard of care or traditional method of care. Clinical trials also help to define the changes required so that older standards can be replaced by more effective ones.

When researchers identify a possibility, they follow stringent guidelines to present and test that possibility. The research must be designed. This includes a definition of what specifically is being tested, who it is being tested on, what existing methods it is compared with, what outcomes are expected, and what the timeline is for patients who will be participating. Although participation is voluntary, there are eligibility requirements to be included in a study, such as:

- age range, general health and gender

- disease type or location, grade, and stage

- prior treatments

- specific qualifications like geography and heredity.

Before the new method is brought forward for trials with patients, it must be successfully tested in the lab. Then, the new method is tried on patients in standard phases as follows:

- <u>Phase I Trial</u>: The treatment is tested on people for the first time. The maximum tolerated dosage and side effects are evaluated. This is called TOXICITY. If unacceptable side effects occur, such as severe liver or kidney damage, the treatment does not advance in trials. Usually, only a small number of patients are involved in these trials, and most have advanced illness where other treatments have failed.

- <u>Phase II Trial</u>: This is comparison testing, designed to reveal whether the treatment is more promising than what is currently available. A Phase II trial involves a small number of patients compared against historical figures instead of a control group.

- <u>Phase III Trial</u>: This phase of testing shows how the new treatment compares to standard treatments. Two groups partake in the study: One group undertakes the new treatment. The other acts as the control and receives the standard treatment. A Phase III trial is a direct comparison of a promising treatment from a Phase II trial with the best current therapy. These trials are usually much bigger, involving more patients in multiple institutions. If a Phase III trial shows a significant difference, then the new treatment becomes standard therapy.

- <u>Introduction to Standard of Care (or sometimes referred to as Phase IV Trial)</u>: If the new treatment passes the trials and is determined to be equal to or better than the current treatments, it is released to more patients in multiple disease states. It is introduced as an equivalent or improved "standard" of care.

People often question cancer research and its findings: They want to know where the money goes and why we haven't yet found a cure. While there are numerous studies happening at any given point, not all of them yield successful outcomes. When a treatment is found to be ineffective on humans or not providing greater benefit than existing methods, the trial may be closed. Or, the research may lose funding or support from sponsoring entities in pursuit of other projects.

Even with studies that are fully funded and come to completion with successful outcomes, it may take years for the devices or medicines to be manufactured and distributed. Additionally, when the clinical trials involve a drug or device, researchers in the United States must submit an application for approval with the Food and Drug Administration (FDA). The FDA must approve the drug or device before it can be marketed. While this extra step is intended to safeguard the public from other undesirable outcomes, it also may add years to getting the medicine to those who need it.

You may wonder how doctors and other medical professionals hear about research that is happening and clinical trials that are running. They learn by reading medical journals when research findings are published and by attending conferences where they are first announced. In the United States, medical professionals must continue their medical education (CME) to maintain their licenses to practice. They earn CME credits by participating in these conferences because current research is discussed that may positively impact their area of expertise. Often, they are provided with status of new treatment approval. Then they know when to offer the treatments to their patients as that approval takes place.

It's important that medical research happens. Medical advances are good for everyone. If the patient is interested in trying a new treatment through participation in a clinical trial, you will need guidance. Ask the patient's oncologist about the rights of participants before you get started. These rights include privacy, informed consent, options to leave the study and options to change treatments or facilities if the study is not right for them.

Benefits of Taking Part of a Clinical Trial

- Clinical trials offer quality cancer care, with the experimental component usually offered for free.

- The patient may have access to a treatment literally years before it becomes available to the general public. The patient will help to shape the future of cancer care and treatment.

- Experimental treatments may offer the possibility of a treatment when no existing traditional treatments are considered effective for the patient's cancer. If the treatment works, the patient may be among the first to benefit and increase his odds of beating the disease or increasing the quality of his life.

Items to Consider When Thinking About a Clinical Trial

- Because these are trials, the outcomes can be uncertain. The patient will not be able to choose if he is in the control group or the new treatment group. There may be side effects that do not surface in earlier phase trials and the patient may need additional medical attention to counter these.

- The trial may be conducted in a location that is geographically hard to reach, although travel costs are sometimes reimbursed for patients and caregivers.

- Health insurance and managed care providers do not always cover all patient care costs in a study, but the studies are usually sponsored in part by another entity.

- These studies require a commitment from the patient and caregiver. The patient and caregiver may need to read through large amounts of information on the trial, including the trial description, potential benefits, and side effects. Clinical trials also mean extra paperwork and time.

A Few Words on Private Research Programs

Private research programs are sometimes available to patients with specific illnesses. In these programs, research is designed for an individual patient's needs. The patient or family pays for the treatment, which is usually administered by the participating or sponsoring doctor. The sponsoring doctor leads the program, and the participating doctor is one of many doctors involved in the program.

In these programs, there may or may not be a control group. You may not have historical data to compare results with, except for the patient's previous condition. These programs are also less stringently monitored. However, the outcomes may be helpful for the patients, as they are designed directly for them. If you're interested in finding out what may be available for the patient in terms of private research, check with the oncologist's office for availability.

Exploring Alternative and Complementary Medicine

"You could tell how much my father really loved my mother when she was diagnosed with breast cancer," said Beth, 28. "My father researched and tried every possible cure and deterrent he could find. He even bought a goat and tied it to a post in the back of the yard so that he could bring my mom fresh goat's milk. He read somewhere that would help. Unfortunately, she was way past the point that anything could help."

We've all seen them – pharmaceutical companies or businesses that promise miracle cures for cancer. You may also have read about natural products that seem to aid the body in fighting specific forms of the disease. Cancer is a very complex family of diseases, and there is no single cure for all types.

To protect the consumer, there are organizations to test and research the reported results of various complementary and alternative practices. These are compared to standard methods and the results of patients who have had no treatments. There is much hope that some of these practices will yield definitive results in fighting the diseases. In the meantime, these sections about alternative and complementary medicines include information to help caregivers understand their care options and make good choices with the patient.

Alternative Therapies

Alternative therapies are conducted *instead of* traditional practices. They replace surgery, radiation, or chemotherapy. Complementary therapies are those conducted *along with* traditional practices, often to compensate for some side effects or to strengthen the effects of the other treatment.

Like Beth's dad in the quote above, some people are so driven in the pursuit of good care that they exhaust all possibilities – usual and unusual – to work towards a miracle cure. Thousands of products, devices, medicines, and food remedies exist for this purpose. There are also dozens of books on natural and holistic healing, usually focusing on diet, emotional states, and environment.

Perceived Benefit of Using Alternative Therapies

Alternative medicines seem to empower the patient and caregiver: they feel they are doing something above and beyond what the normal recommendations for care would be. Caregivers report that they feel as though they are adding to the suggestions from the medical professionals.

Items to Consider

- When you are planning treatment, remember that alternative treatments are not always painless and they may detract from the effectiveness of a traditional approach. Using them may risk a delay of proven treatments.

- Only a small number have been tested. Even fewer have been found to be effective in limiting the occurrence of cancer. Much to our dismay, none have been found to get rid of it altogether.

Research is currently being conducted by major universities and hospitals to provide alternatives for future care. After this research is conclusive, this book will be revised to include those options as viable treatment.

Complementary Therapies

Complementary therapies are different from alternative therapies because their purpose is to complement, or *add to*, traditional treatments. These include products like supplements, foods and extracts. They also include movements and methods to encourage changes in metabolism as the body restores a balance. These can be considered for use before, during and after treatments. Many people believe that the positive impact of traditional therapies can be increased and the negative side effects can be decreased through complementary therapies.

Benefit of Using Complementary Therapies

- Complementary therapy has been used to ease some symptoms from the flu, indigestion, or the common cold. In cancer patients, symptoms including nausea, vomiting, constipation, diarrhea, indigestion, cold sores, cramping, and insomnia often can be eased in a natural way. An example of this is drinking prune juice (which may be less harsh on the system than some medicines) to counter constipation.

Items to Consider

- Be careful of claims without research. Look for statistics and testimonies that can be questioned and verified – like alternative therapy, there are many that may do more harm than good.

- Some of these therapies have not been studied. They may have side effects of their own – including effects on the immune, cardiovascular, or musculoskeletal systems.

With any treatment, remember we highly recommend that you to ask your doctor before starting any complementary practices. If you decide to investigate homeopathic, naturopathic, herbal or aromatherapy options, involve a professional in that field to increase the likelihood of intended results. You can probably find someone on the internet or in a phone book. Ask as many questions as you have and be sure to see if this care is covered by your insurance policy.

Avoid being persuaded to use these approaches based only on patient testimonials or experience. Ask for results of clinical trials published in an industry journal, which will show that it is likely to be more safe and effective.

Helping the Patient Decide on Treatment

> *"They say that chemotherapy after the surgery is 'optional,'"*
> *says Brett, 24, whose mother is fighting pancreatic cancer.*
> *"I would think everyone would want to do that, to make sure*
> *it's all gone."*

You've successfully gotten through the really tough medical material at the front of this chapter – Good job. Our next step is to help the patient decide on a treatment approach. By now, you may have a good understanding of what you think the patient should do. But if you're not clear or if the patient is undecided, discuss your options together. Choosing a treatment approach can be overwhelming and it should not be up to you to make those decisions, unless you have been designated with Healthcare Power of Attorney for her.

It is important that the patient actively participate in care decisions – it is, after all, her life. However, if the patient does not want to take an active role in researching or making her care decisions, she doesn't have to, but she must be given the option. Remind her that she doesn't have to have treatment and that she can always change her mind before treatment starts.

One way to help the patient decide on treatments is to take these steps together:

Step 1: Collect the information on treatment options. If you haven't had a chance to research them, it's OK. Look at what you have, which may only be the recommendations of the doctor, and that's OK.

Step 2: Identify what the patient wants from the treatment. There are several items that could guide her choice. She could rely on response rate alone to make her decision. Response rate is the percentage of people with the same type of cancer who have had a favorable response to a particular course of treatment in the past (basically, how well it has worked). That's important. However, there are other factors, like the impact to fertility or the financial burden of what's not covered by insurance. Still others consider pain, discomfort, and quality of life. Talk about these things, and try to rank them by importance. If one factor is important, it may eliminate an option or steer you towards another.

Step 3: Compare the possible good outcomes of the treatment options with what you want. Set realistic expectations after talking to the patient's medical professionals.

Step 4: Compare the not-so-good possible outcomes, such as side effects, with what you want. Some medical personnel describe this as a risk-benefit ratio. Again, have realistic expectations about what you will be facing. Unfortunately, it's not all good. But if it will save a life, you may want to consider it.

Making treatment decisions is probably not going to be easy. It may take some patience to get used to the idea of having treatment in the first place. Next, we'll look at some reactions that you may see in the patient during this emotional process.

Anticipating Common Patient Reactions

Cancer often holds the top spot on the list of Biggest Threats to a Relationship. While your relationship to the patient may not have been a bed of roses before the DIAGNOSIS, it may not improve now. Treatment is challenging on every level. To get through it, there must be an understanding between you: Cancer is the enemy – fight the cancer, not each other.

This may mean, unfortunately, that you will need extra tolerance. You may have concerns about the treatments, but they are secondary to the patient, as she is experiencing them first-hand. You may have disagreements about treatments, but unless she has given you Healthcare Power of Attorney, her voice trumps yours every time. This may be challenging, even maddening. There may be points where her reasoning doesn't sound logical or her emotions seem unfounded. Tread lightly. Remember how you felt about her before the cancer.

You may encounter a variety of objections. But try to keep some perspective. Think about this if the roles were reversed. You would likely have some concerns as well.

We've categorized common patient and caregiver concerns like this:

- Personal/Emotional Concerns

- Fertility Concerns

- Work Concerns

- Insurance/Financial Concerns

- Religious Objections to Medical Care.

Let's take a look at each category individually. In addition to reading these, you may want to talk to other cancer survivors and their caregivers to hear the way they've dealt with these concerns. There are many ways that you can decrease the negative reactions and increase the positive ones. That's what we're trying to do here.

Personal/Emotional Concerns

Even though the patient may hear what the medical professionals are recommending, he may not want to follow through with a particular treatment for purely "personal" reasons. Here's a scene for discussion:

You're at the kitchen table with the patient. You're having a cup of coffee, trying to digest what you've just heard: the patient needs treatment and the doctor suggests a specific next step. You're supposed to call and set up an appointment at the soonest possible date. The patient seemed agreeable at the office, but now, back at home, the patient's true feelings come out, in comments like these:

> "I don't want more brain surgery. I just don't want to go through that again."

> "They say to have radiation for 'palliative' reasons. I'm not sure what palliative even means."

> "I'm 80. Why do I need chemo? I've had a full life."

> "I'm not going to ask my sister for her bone marrow. We haven't spoken in years and I don't need a transplant that badly."

It may be quite difficult to put emotions aside – for you and her. Many of the emotions like fear, anger, and resentment are easy to empathize with. Still, they may be surprising when they seem to be opposite what the patient expressed in the doctor's office. You have the difficult job of deciding how you want to acknowledge them.

You and the patient may choose to have the treatment as recommended, delay the treatment, or not have any treatment at all. The best course of action is to listen and support the patient's wishes. You may want to involve a therapist, a social worker or the oncologist's nurse if you need a professional to work through the issues.

Fertility Concerns

Protecting the ability to have a child is a high priority for many people. The processes involved in conceiving, carrying, and delivering a child are complex. They involve many glands, organs, and hormones. The timing and environment have to be right for a healthy child to be born. It's easy to see why it's often referred to as a miracle.

Both cancer itself and the treatments to combat it can negatively impact any part of fertility. Men and women in child-bearing years have had compelling concerns for not having treatment:

> ➤ "After the surgery, the doctor says I may need a penile implant. Is it worth it to have to wear one of those the rest of my life?"

> ➤ "They're telling me to have two other procedures: One to move my ovaries up by the kidneys and one to move 'em back after radiation. What if they don't get put back right?"

> ➤ "I just want to finish out this pregnancy before I start chemo. I know I'm sick, but I don't want the chemo to affect the baby."

Put simply, if you are advised that the treatment may make the patient sterile or infertile, you have the same four options as any other cancer patient: to proceed, to wait on it, to elect a less threatening treatment, or to elect the option of no treatment. If your concerns continue, however, here are some suggestions:

- Ask your doctor to refer you to a fertility specialist for another opinion. Get a consultation on your exact issues, whether they are challenges in the male, the female, or both. The specialists will help you navigate your options.

- There are many options to safeguard healthy cells to try for later pregnancy.

  o If you are interested in freezing sperm, do some research to find reputable clinics and sperm banks.

  o If you are interested in protecting eggs, ask your oncologist. Unfertilized eggs can be protected using hormone therapy to prevent their release. The unfertilized egg storage process has not been perfected and is not usually recommended. However, fertilized eggs can be frozen (embryo cryopreservation) and later transferred back into the uterus of the female with much success. This procedure, called in vitro fertilization (IVF), can cost $10,000 or more but the outcome may be worth the cost.

- Ask about ovarian tissue freezing and transplantation. This technology allows the ovary tissue, like fertilized egg and sperm, to be frozen outside of the woman's body and re-planted for later use.

- Ask about infertility surgery. Abnormalities resulting from treatment, such as blockage, polyps or scar tissue, may be overcome with infertility surgery, to increase the potential of reproduction.

Whatever you decide, keep every one of the medical professionals on the patient's case informed of your wishes. This is critical as the patient is considering treatment options, during treatment, and post-treatment. These medical professionals can work in tandem, address your concerns, and offer suggestions to safeguard fertility.

Work Concerns

Although having treatment for a serious illness is important, it is sometimes outranked by work concerns. You may hear job-related concerns stretching into decision-making for care, like:

> ➤ "I'm the breadwinner. I cannot afford to stop working for a little surgery. My family needs the money and not more expenses."

> ➤ "Radiation for 25 days straight? No way. I'm up for a big promotion and now is not the time to be away from the office. This job is my life."

> ➤ "I've been a truck driver almost all my life. If I can't do this job because I'll be all chemo'd up, I'm worthless."

> ➤ "Our family owns this business. If people in our little town found out about the cancer, they might be afraid. We'd be shut down. Better to act 'business as usual' and not take any time off."

If you or the patient is working, you are undoubtedly thinking about how the treatment or series of treatments will affect your job. A job represents many things to people: not only is it their financial security, it may be their link to insurance benefits and it is part of who they are as a person.

A diagnosis of cancer can change all of that. The fact is that doctor appointments take time, generally during business hours. It consumes mental and physical energy. It threatens income-earning potential and generates expenses. Because of this, work is one of the major areas of concern when discussing treatment options.

And these are valid concerns. It's likely there will be missed work, problems with attention, and fatigue, all of which lead to unfulfilled responsibilities. Unfortunately, promotion and recognition can be affected as well: you aren't there, you're not doing the work, and it's been given to someone who was. You may even lose your job if you're not there to do it.

It's difficult to say that the employer is wrong for rewarding employees that are at work accomplishing their objectives without special needs or wanting time off. They're not. Employers should, however, extend flexibility and understanding when these types of situations do surface. Flexibility and fairness are not always present on the job, though. Discrimination does happen, both because an employee faces a serious illness and because an employee is a caregiver of a person with a serious illness.

When evaluating your situation, act within the limits of the company. Find out what reasonable accommodations are available, such as time off, a reassignment, or job flexibility. This may help you make the treatment and timing decisions.

Before you and the patient schedule treatment, check into the Family and Medical Leave Act (FMLA), the Americans with Disabilities Act (ADA), and the Federal Rehabilitation Act (FRA) of 1973. These acts will be useful to both patients and caregivers as they need time for treatment, recovery, and training for new responsibilities. A synopsis of each is included here.

Family and Medical Leave Act

The Family & Medical Leave Act was signed into law in 1993 to allow people to take time away from work to care for their families or themselves. This federal Act allows people who work for companies that employ more than 50 people to take up to 12 weeks of unpaid leave a year to care for a newborn or newly-adopted child, or for certain seriously ill family members (parent, child or spouse). Under the Act, the patient is also covered to recuperate from his own serious health conditions. Some benefits administrators call this the 12-12-12 rule. If the employee has worked at the company for at least 12 months and has worked at least 1250 hours during that period, he could be entitled to take up to 12 weeks unpaid leave.

Both patient and caregiver are covered and therefore, their jobs and related insurance will be secured for this time. The leave, however, is unpaid, which allows the companies to pay another person to take over the responsibilities of the vacating person. However, you and the patient must give written notice to explain the cause of your leave and what dates are applicable, so the employer has enough time to plan for the absence. Those taking advantage of this Act must also report periodically on their status, to allow the employer time to prepare for any changes.

Americans with Disabilities Act

Under this Act, discrimination of people with handicaps or impairments is prohibited. This means that the patient may not be denied a job, promotion, new responsibilities, or pay because of the experience with cancer. Therefore, if the patient needs to find a new job after diagnosis, he is protected from discrimination.

In addition to the ADA and FMLA, there may be state laws or union contracts that enable you to have a greater leave time with job protection. Other caregivers have also reported that they were able to facilitate individual agreements between patient and company or caregiver and company over a short period of time during or just after treatment. Some of these examples are job-sharing, part-time work, flex hours, or a change in responsibilities.

Federal Rehabilitation Act

The Federal Rehabilitation Act applies to entities that are funded by the federal government. Individuals with physical and mental disabilities may approach state entities for assistance searching for and securing meaningful and gainful employment and independent living. You may want to call the Department of Labor in the state where the patient resides for more options on employment, training, compensation, and benefit information.

Cancer can demand an incredible amount of time, energy, and financial resources. You have to address the patient's concerns and your own. Do not rule out the possibility that you or the patient can continue working or return to your jobs after dealing with this. Do not rule out the idea that your current employer(s) would be willing to help you out – in fact, many have experienced this personally and will be more than happy to be flexible. The important things are to keep them informed, make every effort to keep true to what you agree to, and be in communication about any changes.

Insurance/Financial Concerns

Insurance and financial concerns are closely associated with work concerns, because most people have insurance policies through their jobs. Patients have worries like these:

> ➢ "I'm NOT having this treatment. I'll be dropped by my insurance company and what will my wife and kids do for coverage?"

> ➢ "This referral or treatment won't be covered by my health insurance. At least I don't think so. I don't even know who to ask."

> ➢ "If it's not covered, who will pay for it? I don't want to spend the rest of my life paying for an operation that costs thousands."

> ➢ "This is partially covered, but I can't even afford to pay the part that's not."

You may have similar concerns as a caregiver. These are very real and they do not go away, especially as the bills begin to pile up. Before you panic, understand what your insurance coverage and financial responsibilities will be with a given treatment option. Those expenses considered Out-of-Pocket costs may include:

- initial consultations, second opinions, or other advice beyond second opinions

- surgical procedures, medical devices, or prosthesis

- deductibles or expenses over the maximum payouts per year

- coverage for experimental treatments

- personal costs, such as transportation to the treatment center.

You'll want to be sure that you can pay for the services your insurance will not cover. Before you make the treatment decisions, review your policies with a benefits administrator.

Religious Objections to Medical Care

In rare circumstances, the patient will have religious reasons for not wanting treatment. Listen to her objections. Try to understand her perspective. Again, be sure that this is the real reason for objecting to the treatment – not just fear. A treatment could save her life. Unless you have been given Healthcare Power of Attorney, though, the decision is up to her.

The Choice of Non-Treatment

When it appears that the risks of a procedure seem to outweigh the benefits or that the patient has strong reasons for not pursuing treatment, then support her. In certain instances, the medical professionals will advise against treatment, especially with those who are elderly, medically fragile, or challenged by multiple health issues (where a patient may lose the fight to other ailment).

It is OK for the patient to "do nothing" to combat the cancer. It is her choice.

However, that doesn't necessarily make it easy for you to deal with, especially if you have encouraged her to undergo one treatment option or another. Many of us want the patient to try everything possible. But it's not our choice. Hard as that may be to hear, it's true. When the patient decides against treatment, realize that there is another choice in front of you: the choice of HOSPICE and PALLIATIVE

CARE (also called comfort care). If you decide to go this route, ask the patient's medical professionals for guidance.

Interacting with the Patient

During this time of unknowns, there will be a series of trials-and-errors. You may not be able to tell how the patient is feeling at any given time. To make things more challenging, the patient may not recognize those feelings either. She may change her mind moment to moment. These failures in communication can be completely frustrating. How do you cope? You keep trying to communicate. Some days it will be easier than others.

What Do I Say? Talking with the Patient

You are the best one to evaluate when to talk and when to listen. When she's ready, bring up subjects that are easy to talk about first, and then bring up those that could be sensitive later. Consider adding in some of these phrases:

- I know you have some fears about appointments coming up. Let's talk about it.

- The doctor gave me some information. Let me walk you though it.

- You seem confused about this. Are the words sinking in OK?

- Are you sure this discussion is helping? Has the doctor's explanation made any impact?

- What do you think about the side effects or risks of the particular treatment?

- Would you like to take another person with you when the treatment happens?

- Lie down and rest. It's OK to relax.

- Don't give up. There's so much to live for.

- I am here for you. Somehow we will get through this!

How Can I Help? Having Others Involved

As part of your interaction with the patient, you'll want to involve others. Whether she admits it or not, the patient needs you and other non-medical members of your Care Team. The opportunities to help her are many, but here are a few quick tips:

- Be a hospital traffic cop for well-wishers. Bring people to visit, like friends or co-workers.

- If the patient has children, bring them in for a visit to the hospital before the patient has an extended stay. Let them see that the place is safe and non-threatening.

- If the hospital allows it, bring in the patient's pet. There's something healing about unconditional love.

The patient may not be able to receive visitors all the time. Nor will he want to talk to every visitor every time, but most of the time he will.

Taking Care of Yourself

Get ready, Caregiver! Preparing yourself for the patient's upcoming treatment is as important (or even more so) as preparing the patient. You may need some armor. You should remember that it's in the patient's best interest to be good to yourself – It means you can continue to give good care. On days that you're tested, you'll be more centered and better equipped emotionally to handle what comes your way. Here is a collection of Do's and Don'ts coming from seasoned caregivers.

Do's

- Carve out one part of each week for something that gives you pleasure: taking a relaxing bath, preparing a great meal, reading a wonderful book.

- Acknowledge your own emotions about this: the biggies are frustration, anger, lack of control, fear, and fatigue. You're only human.

- Keep flexibility in your routine. You should always expect things to change at any time.

- Encourage yourself every day. Remind yourself why you're doing this. It could be love, a promise or an obligation. Every reason is a good one.

- Give thanks. It could always be worse.

Don'ts

- Don't worry about your skills as a caregiver. Doing something wrong can happen to anyone. Respect your own capabilities and be confident in your approach.

- Don't pretend that you don't have needs, or that you know how to handle everything.

- Don't promise to do everything today. Use procrastination as a tool; sometimes people will step in to help or the need will go away with time. Take care of the critical items first and those smaller things will sometimes take care of themselves.

You're making really important decisions about your life and the patient's life. Keep going – you can do this.

Wrapping Up

You've read through some very scary and scientific information.

In this chapter, we've talked about:

- The traditional treatments of cancer. These are surgery, radiation, and chemotherapy. Treatments are also called therapies or modalities. They can be used separately or together for the patient's benefit.

- Other treatment options. These include alternative and complementary therapies, participation in clinical trials and private research programs.

- Personal and work-related objections to having treatment.

While it's hard to remember all of it, try to remember these few things: You and the patient have choices in treatment options. Unless you have been given Healthcare Power of Attorney, though, it is the patient's right to choose. It's up to the patient whether to have treatment and if so, which type(s).

Don't be afraid to refer back to specific sections if you need to review them again. It's a lot to take in. If you and the patient decide not to pursue traditional treatment, talk to your medical professional about hospice and palliative care (comfort care). If you and the patient decide that pursuing treatment is your best option, keep reading. The next chapter will help you prepare for treatments by describing typical appointments and providing checklists to make things go more smoothly.

Chapter 5: Preparing with the Patient for Treatment

"My husband got a little packet from the oncologist about the procedure," says Lisa, 50. "Is there anything that I can use to prepare myself?"

Whether you know it or not, you've already begun preparing with the patient for treatment. You've been with him in the doctor's office and heard medical recommendations. You've made the decision on treatment types. Now you'll need to know how to manage the upcoming appointments. The goal of this chapter is to familiarize you with what happens during typical treatment scenarios and give you suggestions on how to reduce the frustration and tension that sometimes comes with them.

We'll talk about:

- Traditional Treatment Appointments

- Patient Care Scheduling and Other Practical Preparations

- The Relationship with Medical Professionals

- Taking Care of Yourself.

This chapter has some medical information in it as well, but we've broken it down to make it easier to read. You made it through the last sections just fine, and you'll be able to understand these, too.

Keep in mind how far you've come. You're getting to be an expert on the patient's illness and care. After the patient has started treatment, it could be a relatively short time in his recovery. So let's get started on these preparations to minimize the bumps along the way.

Reviewing Typical Treatment Scenarios

"After we heard it was prostate cancer, we really went into action," says Marla, 65. "In fact, we prepared more for his surgery than my delivery of our three children. We read the doctor's literature. We reviewed our surgery coverage. As best as we could, we figured out what we needed to do, then we got other people involved. Everyone had a little assignment. When it actually came time for the surgery, we were ready."

While each patient situation is different, there are some consistencies in the treatment experience. The patient will go through a series of appointments, depending on the treatment. These are:

1. Consultation

2. Review and scheduling of the procedure

3. SIMULATION (for radiation only)

4. NEOADJUVANT THERAPY

5. Procedure

6. Recovery in the healthcare setting.

Each of the scenarios is described below, starting with Consultation. You will see information specific to treatment types under each heading. Read what is relevant to the type of treatment you are pursuing. Take a deep breath. This will be over before you know it.

Consultation

At this point, you've probably already had necessary consultations to decide your treatment approach, but we'll review it just in case you need to meet with other specialists.

All doctors are not skilled in all treatments. One doctor may consult with another doctor/specialist if the patient's case requires it. After the patient is referred by another doctor, he will meet with the trained specialist. Usually, this is a general surgeon or surgical oncologist for surgery, radiation oncologist for radiation, or oncologist for Chemotherapy. That professional will examine the patient and review all relevant patient records or scans. As the specialist makes the assessment, he may order more tests before recommending next steps.

How to Prepare

Preparing for this appointment is the same for most treatment types. Schedule the appointment as soon as you can. Make sure that the specialist has all the patient's medical records. Either send them ahead or bring them with you. Often, x-rays and other scans can be emailed or put onto CDs for easy transport. Research the patient's disease to have a little familiarity with the terms the specialist may use. Be early for the appointment. You may have to wait, but be ready if you don't. Bring a pad of paper with your questions already written. If you have questions about fertility, bring up them up early. Bring a pen to jot things down or a recorder to use in the conversation.

Review and Scheduling of the Procedure

The review and scheduling of the procedure may be included in your consultation. The specialist will explain the recommended approach to the procedure, preparation and timeframes. He will go over SURVIVAL RATES and set expectations on the patient's response, including SIDE EFFECTS and possible complications. Then, the specialist will review other options for treatment. After the decision to have treatment is made, he will provide ways to schedule it.

Surgery: He will also discuss any short or long-term changes in functioning.

Radiation: He will also discuss the general location of administration and the doses. The radiation oncologist will go over the preparation, or setup, where the exact field of treatment will be determined in a simulation.

Chemotherapy: He will also cover the administration, agents and doses.

How to Prepare

Keep taking notes. You may have to learn to write quickly! Ask for some time to discuss the options, as well as the name of a survivor or a support group with whom you can discuss the treatment. After you and the patient have decided to pursue this option, ask for recommendations on what the patient should do to be physically ready for the treatment.

Bring your calendars and plan the next treatment or appointment as a priority over other items. If there is a gap in treatments, it may alter the effectiveness of the treatment. Be sure to understand when the patient can be transported and what home care needs will be. Get a contact number for problems between visits, such as the nurse, nurse practitioner, or office manager. Take a practice trip to the facility before the first treatment. This will help you understand where you need to be and what obstacles you need to avoid.

Surgery: Be sure to talk about the anticipated effects of the anesthesia and the time of recovery. If the patient's procedure will involve something you're not familiar with, ask questions about it.

Radiation: Sometimes for bladder, prostate, or pelvic treatments, it may be recommended that the patient have the treatments with a full bladder. Ask if this is appropriate for the patient's situation. Discuss your physical contact with the patient after treatment because of skin sensitivities.

Chemotherapy: If the doctor says there will be temporary hair loss, ask for a prescription for a "cranial prosthesis for ALOPECIA." This way, if you decide to purchase a wig, it is more likely to be covered by insurance.

Simulation

This appointment applies only to radiation. It may take several hours to precisely determine the treatment field and intensity. The patient is normally asked to lie still beneath an x-ray machine, CT SCAN, or other imaging machine. Then the medical professionals define the areas that need to be treated, as well as those that need to be shielded. The area is marked or tattooed on the skin of the patient. This tattoo consists of five or six dots drawn with semi-permanent ink. For later treatments, this ensures that the area is consistent and the patient does not have to repeat the location process each time. It's important to not rush this activity, because an accurate marking increases the success of the treatment and decreases severe impacts to vital organs.

How to Prepare

Tell the patient to leave valuables (like wallet, jewelry, or handbag) at home and to wear comfortable clothing. Bring a sweater or a light jacket, as the waiting rooms are often kept cool. Ask the radiation oncologist if there are suggestions or recommendations about eating before and after the radiation. Take books (including this one), crossword puzzles, magazines, or other work to pass the time while you are waiting for the patient.

Neoadjuvant Therapy

You may remember that neoadjuvant therapy is therapy used prior to another treatment. These therapies are prescribed to increase the effectiveness of another treatment type. As an example, radiation may be administered pre-surgery to shrink or stop the cancer TUMOR from growing before it can be removed.

How to Prepare

See the specific sections for treatment preparation. Also, review the doctor's recommendations, including prescriptions. Fill them as appropriate. If you know your local pharmacist or can request a pickup time, do so, so you'll have a shorter wait. As much as possible, get plenty of rest before the appointment (both of you!). Leave early so that if there are unexpected delays, the patient's treatment is not postponed or cancelled for the day – it could throw off the entire treatment calendar.

Procedure

The procedure for each type of treatment is unique.

Surgery: The patient will be given anesthesia in one of three ways: local, IV sedation or general. After the patient is numbed or asleep, an incision will be made where the surgery will take place. Depending on the purpose of the surgery, cells will be removed and then the surgeon will reconstruct the operative site. If there are multiple surgeries happening one after another (such as breast RECONSTRUCTION after a MASTECTOMY), they usually take longer than a single operation and may require additional healing time.

Radiation: The patient will be asked to lie down, and she may have custom molds or masks for optimal immobilization. The rays will be given from multiple angles. The beds may move or the machine may rotate. The patient will know when the radiation has started or finished by the click of machine. It takes between 5-30 minutes, and is normally given daily for 10-40 days, depending on the intent of treatment. If the patient has IMPLANT or Brachytherapy, you can prepare by looking at the suggestions for surgery.

Chemotherapy: This will probably take place in a clinical setting, with the patient in bed or reclining chair and a television at her disposal. The chemotherapy is given by IV or injection. This can take minutes or hours, depending on the PROTOCOL. After this, the patient can usually return home when the treatment is finished. With later appointments, blood may be given to keep up adequate BLOOD COUNTS.

However, the patient may take chemo orally (by pill) at home, like other prescriptions. In this case, be sure the patient follows the instructions on the label, especially in terms of eating and drinking.

How to Prepare

For every treatment, suggest that the patient follows the same advice as preparing for a Simulation: Leave valuables (like wallet, jewelry, or handbag) at home, and wear comfortable clothing. Bring a sweater or a light jacket, as the waiting rooms are often kept cool. Ask about the usual length of time for the procedure so you can plan accordingly.

Surgery: Read all materials given to you by the specialist and staff. If there are any pre-op instructions, like fasting or bowel prep, have the patient follow them to the letter. It will make the procedure smoother.

Radiation: It's important for the patient to be in the best possible shape before a procedure, including her skin. So, it would be helpful if you encourage the patient to drink a lot of water (more fluids than normal) and to avoid time in the sun or tanning bed before treatments. Ask about taking care of the skin around the radiated area. If you have been given advice on a healthy diet, follow it with the patient. Both of you should get plenty of rest. It's extremely difficult to dedicate driving and care time for the better part of the month without taking a break. Designate a backup person as a driver or someone who can be with the patient post-treatment, in case another emergency arises.

Chemotherapy: Encourage the patient to go to the dentist to have a teeth cleaning and cavities filled before treatment. If the oncologist says there will likely be temporary hair loss, her head can get cold, so buy hats, scarves, or head wraps. Consider shopping for a wig and wig liner. Get a professional to cut the wig. Place a hand-vacuum near the bed or in the bathroom for easy pickup of hair. If it's approved by the oncologist, discuss exercise of some kind with the patient – even walking in the house – to reduce nausea.

Recovery in the Healthcare Setting

The patient's recovery will depend on the treatment, of course. The medical professionals in the healthcare setting will be the immediate care providers for a certain length of time after the treatment (post-treatment). They will monitor the patient's reactions and manage any complications that arise. When the patient is ready, they will also prepare her for discharge and provide home care instructions.

Surgery: The surgical oncologist or surgeon will review the PATHOLOGY REPORT for more information about the tumor. He will oversee the patient's healing in the hospital and schedule follow-up care upon release.

Radiation: The radiation oncologist will compare the status of the cancer before and after the treatment to validate that the protocol is working. The doctor may change areas, doses, or frequency if the therapy does not appear to be working as it should.

Chemotherapy: The oncologist will compare the status of the cancer before and after the treatment to validate that the protocol is working. As with radiation, the doctor may change agents or timing if the therapy does not appear to be working as it should.

How to Prepare

In general, listen to discharge instructions, even if you already have been told what to do. It can't hurt to hear them again. Gather insurance questions and paperwork together and schedule some time with the office manager or social worker on the same day as the treatment so that you don't have to make two trips.

Surgery: Many procedures require a hospital stay following surgery (post-operatively). If you know the patient will be in the hospital, pack a little care package of pajamas, slippers, magazines, and toiletries so their stay feels a little more like home. Find out visiting restrictions (for adults, children and pets) in different areas of the hospital. If you want to talk to the doctor, call his office and find out when he is making rounds. Have one person be the main point of contact in the family, so that every family member does not ask the same questions.

Radiation and Chemotherapy: The initial patient care following treatment will be handled by the medical professionals until the patient is sent home.

That's it! We understand it's a lot of information, but now you have an overview of the whole six-part process of treatment and ways to prepare. Sometimes, this treatment process doesn't run in a straight line, especially if there are multiple treatment types or complications. But at least you know what's ahead in the overall scheme of things.

As we said previously, you've probably passed Consultations and are ready to proceed with planning treatment. Here is a checklist to guide you.

Scheduling Medical Care for the Patient

You've decided to pursue the course of treatment that will best help the patient. When it's time to call for the treatment appointment, here are a few things you can do to limit your frustration. Make the most of your time on the phone and in the office by following this list.

Checklist: Making Appointments

☐	Work with the medical professionals on the treatment timeline. They will guide you on how immediate the need is.
☐	Bring your calendars and plan the next treatment or appointment as a priority over other items.
☐	Be realistic about timeframes for procedures. Understand what 20 minutes really means – it could be that the radiation dose takes that long, but you actually need to allot two hours for travel time, checking in, dressing, and post-procedure activity.
☐	Get clear instruction on how to complete any prescribed exams, tests, or lab work that needs to be done before the treatment.
☐	Ask whomever you are scheduling the appointment with what you need to bring for each appointment. This may include medical reports, radiographic materials (x-rays, CT or other scans), lab reports from routine tests, and anything else that could help the medical professional to make decisions. If possible, get those materials to the doctor before your visit so he can review them if he has time before the appointment.
☐	If the patient has back-to-back procedures, allow for time to travel between locations. When possible, do a test run between treatment locations to find out how long it will take. Be sure not to schedule so close that you are late.
☐	Be patient. Remember, all the people in the waiting areas have problems, usually equal to or greater than yours. If the doctor or other specialist is behind schedule, understand that he is giving another patient much needed care and you will be given the same courtesy when your turn comes.
☐	Encourage the patient to be responsive to the staff and to follow their instructions.
☐	Many facilities have patient representatives. When possible, meet them. These people are here to help you.
☐	Remember to be polite to office staff members. They often work long hours and they are normally not highly paid. They may be able to work you into a tight schedule or surprise you with a much-needed cup of coffee.
☐	Thank the people involved in the patient's care.

Cultivating Relationships with Medical Professionals

The medical professionals involved in the patient's care are your partners. They will work to address concerns, provide information, and involve specialists as necessary. They take their professions very seriously and they want you to take interactions with them seriously. You need to cultivate a good working relationship with them. That's not to say you can't smile or laugh. You can continue a positive, results-oriented relationship with the medical professionals if you provide them with:

- Accurate MEDICAL HISTORY, including treatment from other doctors

- Truthful answers about any complementary and alternative therapies (even vitamins) that the patient is trying

- Reports on the responses to treatment, as well as any associated symptoms.

Additionally, get to know the names of the nursing staff. No one likes to be called "Hey You" or "Excuse Me." This may be a little challenging, with shift changes three times a day and weekend-only personnel, but it's worth the personal touch they may give back.

Remember, this is a partnership, and if you treat each other well the experience can be a little more pleasant. Caregivers like you have discovered shortcuts that may be helpful in making your time around a medical setting a little more comfortable. Several are contained in the next two checklists.

Checklist: Practical Suggestions INSIDE the Medical Setting

☐	Understand the hours and rules of the care facilities. Read any literature about the hospital relationships and obligations.
☐	Ask if multi-day parking passes are available, and if so, at a discount.
☐	Inquire about a shuttle bus or golf cart from the parking lot, and wheelchairs to use when inside the facility.
☐	Pick up a map of the hospital campus, including tunnels or skywalks to protect you and the patient from the weather. Get familiar with shortcuts between facilities, if any.
☐	Find a lounge where couches or chairs are available.
☐	When the patient is checking in, ask when you can join the patient and when you can't.
☐	If the patient needs to stay for an extended time, ask about room choices. You and the patient may have choices about the room (such as private or semi-private rooms, private bath, room with window by bed, television or music options). If so, decide that early and politely relay your request.
☐	Understand what you may bring into the patient's room. These can include clothing, music, photos, reading materials, or toiletries.

Checklist: Practical Suggestions OUTSIDE the Medical Setting

☐	Go to the restroom before heading over to an appointment. You may have long waits, be far away from restrooms, or you may be unable to leave the patient.
☐	Don't schedule things immediately after treatment. You won't be able to estimate the reactions of the patient, nor the potential delays.
☐	Find pharmacies that stay open long hours, so when you need them you know where to go.
☐	Cook meals in advance and freeze foods in meal-size portions; cut veggies or bring crackers to snack on. You won't feel like cooking coming home from treatment. You may not feel like eating, but if you do it will be simple to heat something up instead of going through the cooking process.
☐	Investigate relaxation techniques if the patient is apprehensive about a procedure.
☐	Look into stretching and flexibility DVDs or tapes or classes that you can take, with or without the patient. Often these are suggested to reduce stiffness and swelling for various kinds of treatment, as well as aid in healing and stress reduction. Check with your medical professionals to be sure this is right for you.

If you need ideas on handling common questions from other people, read on.

What Do I Say? Talking to Others about the Patient's Progress

There is one consistency in the caregiving process: other people will not know what comments to make or questions to ask. With differing levels of appropriateness, it is difficult to determine what is welcome conversation and what is better left unsaid. Many people will have an interest in the patient's well-being, but it may not surface in a caring way. In fact, it may come out as somewhat judgmental, abusive, or unfeeling. Dealing with upcoming cancer treatment is not an everyday occurrence for any of us and it's not easy.

Sensitivities will surface when you're preparing for treatment and as treatment begins. Try to realize that most people are doing what they believe is best. They just may not know better. Use the unknowns and discomforts to your advantage. You can be the gatekeeper to the information that you know, sharing what you want, when you want. Your audience will probably understand. Try these answers:

- **"How is the patient?"** – To those who inquire in a heart-felt fashion, answer in a way that invites support, like "We're really scared, but encouraged. She starts treatment tomorrow and I know she would love to hear from you afterwards." To those who seem disingenuous or who bring discomfort to you or the patient, you can respond with an honest but vague answer like "Thanks for asking. We're working with the medical professionals and we're waiting to see what will happen next."

- **"Why didn't you consult me before letting Mom schedule radiation?"** – Usually, family members or out of town guests who are suddenly interested in the patient's care have limited or no knowledge of the process that led to the decision. If they were not involved in the care before, they have no voice now, especially when time is of the essence and arguing only delays activity. Be firm and satisfied with the treatment choices you have made with your mom (or whomever) based on the information and medical advice you have been given. This may be the first of many episodes of setting limits with those who may not really care, have other agendas, or are not dependable. It will be tough but you can do it.

- **"I've heard of new treatments (new drugs or devices, special healing guru in India, or herbal remedies) that may help."** – How do you respond to unsolicited advice? Maybe consider the advice and the source. Has this person given good advice before? Does the suggestion seem to have merit? If so, consider researching it through articles, brochures, or the internet. In dealing with some overzealous (but well-meaning) people, there may come a point when you need to politely decline information. Explain that "We've made some decisions with our Care Team and developed our Care Plan, but thanks anyway for your suggestions."

Taking Care of Yourself

"I kept waking up every two hours before important appointments, worried that I would miss them," says Charlotte, 37. "I finally tried this crazy remedy. I set two alarm clocks. Then, I put warm water in my bathtub, about two inches high, and march around in it for a few minutes. I get out, dry off and put fuzzy socks on before returning to bed. It works like a charm. I sleep through the night."

We've said throughout this book that it's important to stay well-rested. You need sleep to heal yourself and rejuvenate yourself for another day of your life and caregiving in the patient's life.

Your best bet is to try to sleep during nighttime hours, but it can be difficult to sleep when you're trying to absorb information and make important decisions. The stress can lead to insomnia or fitful sleeping, leaving you sleep-deprived. Chances are, you don't have time to take a much-needed nap during the day, either.

If you're interested in improving your sleep or fighting insomnia, try these tricks used by fellow caregivers:

- Don't watch the news or read disturbing medical material before you try to sleep.

- Avoid caffeine, alcohol or other substances that may keep you awake. Drink warm milk instead.

- Take a warm shower before resting.

- Make the room as dark and quiet as possible.

- Wiggle your toes, and concentrate on them instead of the many other things on your mind.

- Listen to nature sounds like water flowing, rain, ocean waves, birds chirping or the wind. If it's possible rely on Mother Nature for these, but if not, borrow some music from the library.

If you're trying these remedies and still not sleeping well, ask your own doctor about a sleep aid. He may have other suggestions for you that are prescription and non-prescription. Remember, you've got to take good care of yourself, which includes getting good rest.

Wrapping Up

You've just gone through the impressive steps of preparing for cancer treatment with the patient. Even though this is not your treatment, you've gone through the planning checklists and instructions. You should pat yourself on the back for figuring out what needs to be done and lending support to the patient. You've been so strong.

As treatment times approach, you may be a little nervous or scared. Try to find some comfort in the caregiver quotes and suggestions. We've been there too, and we know that your mental health and physical health can be challenged in this process. We want to keep you healthy and you'll need to stay as rested as possible.

The next chapter is dedicated to common activities during treatment, so that you know what to expect and can address them with confidence.

Chapter 6: Maintaining Your Sanity During Treatment

"The ceiling in this waiting room has approximately 63,360 little holes in it," says Doug, 70. "I counted them. Wasn't much else to do. I counted all the holes in that one tile over there, then I counted the number of tiles and multiplied. So, I kind of cheated. But, I'll probably be able to tell you the exact number of holes in a few weeks when all my wife's treatment is through."

When the appointment for the first treatment arrives, there's no more denying it: *the patient really does have cancer.* This often triggers feelings of uncertainty: Are we making the right treatment choices? Will the treatment actually cure the cancer? and How much treatment will the patient need?

It's normal to feel jittery before the first treatment. As treatments begin, you and the patient may share thoughts on how well they are working and the SIDE EFFECTS you are facing. However, if you try to analyze all possible outcomes before the treatments begin, you can lose your mind to worry.

The goal of this chapter is to help you to keep your thoughts straight during the patient's treatment process. We'll walk through what's likely to happen as you:

- Plan Your Trip to the Treatment Facility

- Play the Waiting Game

- Accompany the Patient to Treatment Appointments

- Bring the Patient Safely Home.

- Take Care of Yourself.

Read this whole chapter if you can. With a little planning and a lot of information, some of those jitters will disappear and your sanity can stay in tact. But, we understand that during treatment, time is scarce.

If you have time to read only one thing in this chapter, it should be the next section, *"Heading to the Treatment Facility"*.

If you have limited time to read, review the next section then jump ahead to those sections that apply to the type of treatment she is having. The explanations will help you see behind closed doors when you can't be with her. Treatment facilities like hospitals, clinics, and doctor's offices can be intimidating. Let's get ready to face the patient's treatment program. Armed with the upcoming information, you'll be empowered to do this.

Heading to the Treatment Facility

> *"I keep telling myself 'The sooner we get there, the sooner it's finished,'" says Miles, 47, whose cousin is facing lung cancer. "Why does there always seem to be so much traffic when we're in a hurry?"*

When you need to make a trip to the treatment facility with the patient, your mind may be going in a thousand directions. It's important to understand what's likely to happen and approach one thing at a time. Let's make sure we cover the basics. Breaking it down, we'll go through planning your trip, making the journey, reaching your destination, and moving from the parking lot to the office.

Planning Your Trip

"It wasn't like we were going to the beach," said Saundra, 37. "But, I tried to make my sister's radiation treatments a little 'fun' by bringing something different each time. I brought little gifts for her like outrageous socks, colorful nail files, plastic rings, or smiley stickers. Nothing really expensive, but she loved them. We agreed she couldn't look in my bag until just after her treatment. It gave her something to look forward to."

The patient's first treatment is an anxious experience for both of you. When the day arrives, there will likely be knots in her stomach and butterflies in yours. Keep those butterflies in a holding pattern, though – there's some groundwork to do.

Before you leave for the treatment facility, be sure you have done these three things:

1. Read and followed the pre-treatment instructions you received from the medical professionals for this treatment.

2. Double-checked that you've packed the items you both need during the visit.

3. Notified your support network that today's the day.

Let's take a look at what each means.

1. You have read and followed pre-treatment instructions.

Most treatments come with a set of instructions. These are given to the patient by a medical professional to guide her before, during, and after her treatment. If she follows these instructions, she'll increase her chances for successful treatment results. If she doesn't, she can delay treatment or impact its effectiveness.

Encourage her to follow the pre-treatment instructions. For example, if the instructions say "The patient cannot eat two hours before treatment," make sure she doesn't eat. No matter how much she complains about hunger pangs, don't give her food. As a compassionate person, you'll want to give in. Instead, reassure her and refocus her attention on why she's not eating. For example, when she says, "Please, I just want something little in my stomach," and begs you to stop for fast food, tell her: "I understand. I'm hungry too! But we'll both eat *after* your treatment. We only have a little while yet until the treatment begins and when we follow the doctor's orders, your recovery will be easier. We want you to get the most of each treatment and to get well faster!" It's not easy to counter these objections, but stay strong. A little willpower from both of you will go a long way.

2. You have packed the items you both need during the visit.

Because they're afraid of forgetting something critical, some caregivers bring everything but the kitchen sink to an appointment. Most of the time, you only need a few of those items, so let's narrow it down. Pack a tote with these essentials:

- directions to the facility, including the exact address, phone number, and a contact name in case you get lost

- patient's current medical records, identification, and insurance information

- materials to pass the time, including a pen and paper to jot things down

- something special that gives you comfort, like a small blanket

- little snacks such as granola bars, crackers, or dried fruit that are easy to carry and to keep fresh.

As we mentioned earlier, you should both leave behind wallets, expensive jewelry, and uncomfortable clothing. You'll want to wear clothes and shoes that will be comfortable when walking, sitting, or standing for extended periods of time. Plan what you're going to wear the night before the treatment.

3. You have notified your support network that today's the day.

Many hands make light work. Tell friends and neighbors that are part of your CARE TEAM when the patient's treatments will start. You'll need extra help as the treatments begin to affect your daily living. When others are informed, they'll have a better idea of how and when they can help.

When the timing is right, ask them to contact the community organizations that extend services during treatment. (This may be before or after the first treatment visit.) You've probably already identified the ones you'd like to take advantage of when you put together your CARE PLAN. If not, ask your friends and neighbors to research a little for you. It's comforting to know that others are ready to help when you and the patient head for this appointment.

Making the Journey

"I finally had to ask our neighbor to drive Eddie to the hospital for his chemo treatments," says Marion, 68. "Sometimes I would be so upset or lost in thought it would be like I was driving on autopilot. I wouldn't even remember the drive. But I would remember my husband howling from the back seat: 'That was a stop sign! Are you trying to kill me before we get there? I'm trying to survive here!'"

Allow plenty of travel time to get to the treatment facility. While it may be a short trip, remember Murphy's Law and expect possible delays. It's always better to be a little early than to rush around.

Getting the patient into and out of the car can be a bit of a challenge, especially if he is weak or nauseous. This is relatively common. When he is not able to move on his own, you'll have to help him. If you haven't had training on how to move a patient, here is a three-step lesson.

Step 1: When moving the patient from a wheelchair into a car, it's important for you to have good footing and balance. Put on the wheelchair brakes. Make sure to position the car where he doesn't have to walk without the wheelchair. When you're ready, open the car door and make sure the seat's clear. Move it back as far as it can go. Try to keep it there for future trips. Talk through the move with the patient, rocking him as you get ready. Agree when he's going to stand and help him up. Have him lean on the car for support. As much as possible, have him guide himself in. If he can't get in on his own, help him to sit down, being careful not to knock his head on the door frame. After he's sitting down, encourage him to move his legs in, if possible. If not, gently bring his legs into the car. Have him decide what's most comfortable, sitting upright or lying down, and accommodate his request.

Step 2: After he's inside the car, the patient may want to discuss the illness and the treatment he's about to face. If he feels like talking, talk. Let him guide the conversation. Understandably, he may be nervous or angry. You may find yourself fighting traffic, but don't find yourself fighting the patient. Remember, the enemy is the cancer. Try not to take what he says personally. For example, when he criticizes you for taking a specific route to the treatment facility, calmly reply: "I think we'll avoid some traffic this way. I'm doing my best to get us there safely."

While you concentrate on your driving, suggest the patient think about the schedule of the treatment. If this is the first visit, remind yourselves about what the medical professionals have told you. For example, "We will be in this room. You're going to experience this. It will probably take this amount of time." If this is a repeat visit, confirm with each other that it will be just like the prior one or talk about changes. Again, if the patient feels like talking about it, do so, but don't push it if he doesn't. Caregivers also recommend bringing a favorite pillow, blanket, or eye mask to help the patient sleep on the way. When he's sleeping, you can relax a little yourself.

Step 3: It's often encouraging to the patient to hear comments like "You're halfway-done!" or "After this, we've only got two to go." Some caregivers suggest talking about how the patient will feel afterwards, like: "You know you may be tired and nauseated for a few days, but the good news is we know how to manage that now." Talking about the appointment may help you both be a little more comfortable in the car.

Reaching Your Destination

"It goes like this: You pull in the parking lot. You find a spot you think is close by, and then it turns out that the parking lot is on the opposite side of the building from where you want to be," says John, 44. "Then, you deal with all the stuff inside like finding a wheelchair, getting your wife situated, filling out forms. By the time treatment is finished you're so fried you can't find the stupid car. But we learned from that. Now we use a shuttle service that makes it easy on my wife to get through the parking garage and helps me remember where we parked."

Many activities happen during a treatment visit. The easiest way to manage them is to concentrate on only one thing at a time. Be sure to accommodate the patient's wishes and abilities too, because planning is most productive when everyone's in agreement.

Moving From the Parking Lot to the Office

If you've had the opportunity to do a trial run to the facility before the appointment for the first treatment, then you probably know the lay of the land. If you haven't, you may find several parking choices in front of you. Parking varies with the size of the care facility. Smaller facilities may offer free parking right out front. Larger institutions may have garages or parking lots with colors or letters to navigate them. A few institutions even offer complimentary valet service. If so, use it. However, most sites do not have valet service in hopes of keeping the entrance unobstructed for ambulances and other vehicles to drop off patients who have difficulty walking.

After you and the patient have arrived safely at the treatment facility, you'll want to park in a spot that's right for you. For some, that spot means the one nearest the office. For others, that spot is near a shuttle service or elevator. When the patient has multiple appointments in one visit, the right spot may be closer to the exit of the second appointment than the first, so that they have less distance to travel afterwards.

You may have to try a couple of spots before you find the best parking area for you. You'll learn some shortcuts each time you go to an appointment. In special circumstances, the doctor may provide a handicap parking pass, which enables you to legally park in the blue spaces. *Do not use these spaces if you do not have permission. You will be towed, fined, or both.* Park there only if you have a pass. When you borrow a pass or another piece of equipment, use it appropriately and then return it. That way, that it will be available if the patient (or another person) needs it in the future.

When you've parked, it's time to get the patient out of the car. If she needs help, reverse the process you followed when you put her in the car. Gently sit her up and bring her legs out first. Help her stand and steady her to begin the walk inside. If you are fortunate enough to have a wheelchair or shuttle available, guide her into a sitting position on the seat and head for the office. Take advantage of all transportation services that are offered to you. They may include shuttle buses, the use of wheelchairs or walkers, and volunteers to show you the way. Don't be afraid to ask for assistance, directions, or a map.

Now that you've reached the care facility, let's look at:

- handling office preparations

- winning the Waiting Game

- understanding the treatment procedure

- managing relationships with medical professionals.

Handling Office Preparations

After you've found your way to the right office, it's time to complete the pre-treatment office preparations (prep). There are two types: new and existing.

New Patient Prep

When the patient is new, she will usually need to provide a picture I.D. and proof of insurance. In addition, she will need to bring current medical reports, records, or scans to the office staff. She'll be given new patient registration forms to fill out, as well as office policy information to read. She'll be asked to sign an Informed Consent for Treatment form for the treatment and to identify who she wants her medical information shared with on Health Insurance Portability and Accountability Act (HIPAA) forms. She may be asked to identify someone to act as a Healthcare Power of Attorney and to record her wishes for life sustaining treatment. Additionally, she may be asked to complete a DO NOT RESUSCITATE (DNR) request.

The stack of forms on the clipboard can be overwhelming. If you're helping with the forms, fill out all the information they request, even if it seems to be duplicate. Don't leave something blank without asking the office staff about it. By filling the forms out neatly and thoroughly, you will avoid treatment delays or having to fill them out again.

Pay attention to the HIPAA forms. By signing them, the patient is allowing critical medical information to be shared with the people she listed. Because you are a primary caregiver, it's important that you are included on these forms. Otherwise, no information about the patient's medical condition will be shared with you. Period. You will need access to her information to help with prescriptions, equipment, treatment status, and general home care, so be sure that your name is on that form.

Many people sign forms without reading or understanding them. Read them and ask the front desk personnel if you have questions. They may have explained something a dozen times, but if it takes thirteen times before you process it, that's OK.

Existing Patient Prep

Once on file, the patient's identity and insurance do not need to be revalidated. Usually, the patient will sign in and give the office copies of any new medical information, like recent blood test results. There will be few (if any) forms to fill out. After you get the routine down, each visit will be less involved. You can concentrate on something else – like how to make good use of those times in the waiting room.

Winning the Waiting Game

> *"I got spoiled being the only one working on this puzzle," says Ida, 77. "Isn't it beautiful, with these big sailing ships? Week after week I'd come in and it would be exactly as I left it. I was making progress on it. Almost felt a part of it. Then I came in last week and someone else was working on it. It was like all my frustration burst loose. I just yelled at her. I mean yelled! How dare she think she could work on MY jigsaw puzzle? I scared the daylights out of that poor girl. Now I'm a little embarrassed, and I sure hope whoever it was she was waiting for is done with their treatment."*

Let's just acknowledge it: Waiting is frustrating and upsetting. As a caregiver, you will find yourself waiting during office visits, treatment delays, and recovery times. Because it can happen during every phase of the treatment process, it seems that waiting is an inescapable struggle.

Like any endurance competition, waiting is an opportunity to win. If you look at it as an opportunity to manage the situation, you will triumph over it. How will you be victorious in this waiting game? With the strategies here, both you and the patient can learn to put this wait time to work *for* you instead of *against* you. Let's take a look at some options.

Strategy #1: Get to know your surroundings.

Most clinical settings are designed with creature comforts for the caregivers in mind. You can spend the time learning your way around the facility. Go on a personal scavenger hunt to locate necessities, such as:

- Water fountain, water cooler or bottled water
- Restrooms
- Coffee, snack machines, restaurants or cafeterias
- Public refrigerators and microwaves
- Patient advocate or social worker
- Resource center

- Lounges with couches, and family areas to bring children
- Map of the facility
- Tunnels or skywalks from one treatment center to another
- Chapel
- ATMs
- Gift shop.

Strategy #2: Make use of the resources in the facility.

You will find various resources at the treatment facilities. In general, hospitals have the greatest variety of services. For example, some hospitals have public computers to check email or surf the internet, with helpful cancer web sites already chosen as "Favorites." Resource centers or on-site libraries in hospitals contain patient and caregiver literature, usually pamphlets and books, in a quiet place to read. Support groups affiliated with a hospital present a variety of caregiver functions. You can either sign up for future events or go to ones that are taking place when you're there.

Wellness centers are known to offer relaxation assistance through yoga, stress management methods, and massage. In doctor's offices, waiting rooms tables are often stocked full of magazines and games for children of many ages: crossword puzzles, jigsaw puzzles, board games, checkers, chess, and playing cards.

Strategy # 3: Bring your own distractions.

Listening to music or watching movies may relax you and distract your mind. Carry in your portable player, but remember to wear earphones. Pack a sketch pad, journal, knitting or other much-loved hobby that can fit into a tote bag. You may find it hard to concentrate on work-related materials, but try reading some lighthearted books or magazines.

Strategy #4: Address the paperwork.

Bring a copy of the patient's current insurance policy. Re-read it. Call the insurance company claims number to reach a person assigned to handle your claim. Talk with your claims representative on a regular basis, so that she will be familiar with the patient's needs. Ask for a few blank forms or learn how to file online. Sometimes, the claims representatives can give you hints to shorten the filing processing. They may also help you to re-file insurance claims if they were wrongfully rejected – especially for coding errors (wrong number listed for services) or incomplete information.

Social workers are on-site in many locations, and they can help you with insurance problems and payment questions. They can also talk to you about other topics including the Americans with Disabilities Act (ADA) for the patient and Family & Medical Leave Act (FMLA). By reviewing these acts with them, you may be able to determine your rights in relation to time off and federal assistance.

Strategy #5: Go for a walk.

The change of scenery may do you good. Take a stroll in the hospital courtyard, walk around the building, or investigate a different floor. Don't worry, you're allowed to leave. Notify the nursing station or front office if you think you'll be gone longer than half an hour.

Strategy #6: Write your news report.

To be a successful caregiver, you must be a good communicator. People will want to know what's happening with the patient and you'll be amazed at the responses you get to patient news. You'll get survivor stories, suggestions, encouragement, and expressions of gratitude. But first you have to reach out.

As children, many of us played the Chinese Telephone game. Remember? In the game, a story was told very quickly to the first person, who whispered it to a friend. That friend whispered it to a third player and the game continued. When the last friend heard the story, she stood up and repeated it. Unfailingly, it was so different from the first story that it caused everyone to laugh.

Dealing with medical news is not a laughing matter, but sometimes humor can help to lighten the situation. For example, one woman talks about her husband's surgery, noting "the side benefit is his weight loss." However, it is important to make sure that the information is correct. The best way to avoid the Chinese Telephone effect is to manage what people hear, when they hear it. In general, people care about the patient and want to know the latest news. But you won't have the time or energy to call and repeat the story a hundred times.

You could just jot down a couple of sentences. If you're interested in doing more to communicate, fellow caregivers have come up with creative ideas to get the information out. One idea is asking a friend to start an email/ phone list and give him a script to distribute to everyone on the list. This will keep the information pretty much the same for all recipients. He can also manage any responses. Another idea is asking a friend to help you create a web site with the script you put together. You can give people the URL (internet address) so they can find it and check on the patient's status at anytime. Email is a great way to receive long-distance support.

Strategy #7: Pray, meditate, or just relax.

The chapel is there for a reason. Go in, sit down. You may find some much-needed peace.

Strategy #8: Make a To Do list.

With so many things on your mind, it's easy forget what needs to be done if you don't write it down. Ask yourself if there are prescriptions to be filled, office people to ask about insurance, literature to bring home or other appointments to set. Maybe you need to go to the grocery store, make some calls, follow up on kids' activities or other work at home. Whatever it is, write it down now, delegate it, or cross it off later.

Strategy #9: Take a friend with you.

During the first few appointments, it may help to bring a friend with you. The friend can offer support and a little distraction. In addition, he can learn the ropes so that when you need a break or a back-up on transportation, he can step in for you. You can show him around, introduce him, and discuss what's happening with the patient. He'll know what to expect and it will comfort you to know that while you're gone, the patient is in good hands.

Strategy #10: Catch up on sleep.

Treatments can sometimes take hours, especially if there are back-to-back procedures. Search out that lounge with a couch. Bring a neck pillow or blanket and catch a few winks. Don't feel embarrassed or self-conscious. You're not the first one and you'll certainly not be the last. If you're a heavy sleeper, tell someone at the desk where you are so that someone can find you and wake you when it's appropriate.

Try any of these strategies, or invent your own. Use whatever works for you. The key is to look at it as an opportunity, instead of a setback.

Understanding Treatment Procedures

Usually, the longest stretches of "wait time" are during the treatments themselves. Most medical professionals advise caregivers to learn about the procedures and treatments that the patient will be experiencing. In fact, they often educate the caregivers on what is happening, how long it will take, and what the likely outcomes will be. In short, they help the caregivers prepare themselves.

Overviews of the three most common treatments – SURGERY, RADIATION, and CHEMOTHERAPY are given in the following pages. These tell what is typically happening to the patient and they also explain what that means for you while the treatment is taking place. Each patient's situation is different, but the process is usually similar per treatment type. If you have specific questions that aren't addressed here, ask the patient's medical professional.

Surgery

"It's a matter of trust, I think, when you see your best friend wheeled in for surgery," says Mary Joe, 58. "You want to jump on that gurney with him. You want to protect him and make sure it goes OK. You have no idea what they're doing in there. I mean, the surgeon explained it to us and I watch E.R., but once they close the doors anything can happen. You just have to leave it up to the professionals."

What is Happening to the Patient

When a patient has surgery, he's in a sterile environment. He'll be asked to remove any clothing that is near the area and put on a hospital gown, if necessary. He will be on an operating table for larger operations or an exam table for smaller surgeries. Usually, there will be anesthesia given to him. This is done in one of three ways: locally (at the site), sedation (to make him drowsy), or general (to put him to sleep). The surgical oncologist, or surgeon, will have access to a variety of tools used in surgery. These include: scalpels (surgical knives), forceps (tweezers), scissors, needles, suture (thread), stapling devices, and suction. Every item to be used in the surgery will be counted. The time the operation begins will be noted.

Prior to the surgery, the surgeon's hands and arms will be washed and sterilized. Surgeons will be dressed in operating gowns. Surgical technicians, anesthesiologists and other professionals assist. Under very bright lights, the surgeon will open the area, remove the TISSUE, and close the area. As mentioned earlier in the chapter, surgical patients will be asked to sign an Informed Consent Form. This allows surgeons to act as they deem necessary in the course of an operation. For example, after the surgery has begun, a surgeon may find new cancerous growth. He will need to make a decision if he should remove it now or in a second operation later.

Typically, surgeons who remove a TUMOR will take an additional rim of the tissue around tumor. This extra tissue is called a MARGIN. The goal of taking this margin is to increase the likelihood of removing the entire tumor.

After the procedure is complete, the incision will be covered with a sterile dressing. The exact finish time will be noted and the surgical tools will be counted again. The amount of blood loss will be documented. All tissue removed from the patient will be carefully collected and taken to the Pathology Department for review. The patient will be wheeled into the recovery room and the surgeon will write the orders to care for the patient. The surgeon will talk to you about the operation, and then create a "dictation" of the procedure itself for the patient's medical file.

What This Procedure Means for You

In a sterile environment, no non-medical personnel are allowed to observe. The surgeon will give you an estimate of how long the operation will take. A member of the operating staff may contact you to let you know how the surgery is progressing. The surgeon or a staff member will tell you where the patient is, when it's OK to see him, and what's next. Have patience – you don't want to rush a surgical team. They may finish right on schedule, a little ahead, or a little behind. Use some of the strategies of Winning the Waiting Game during his surgery and while he's in recovery.

Radiation Therapy

"I didn't hear anything going on in there," says Fred, 60. "Has her radiation started yet?"

What is Happening to the Patient

A patient undergoing radiation will be in a room by herself. As with surgery, she'll be asked to remove any clothing that is near the area to be radiated and to put on a hospital gown, if necessary. The precise area of radiation will be determined prior to this visit in a SIMULATION. In this simulation, the patient will be marked with a tattoo or given markings to align the radiation unit to the treatment area.

The patient will be asked to sit or lie down under body molds. These body molds will shield her healthy areas from the radiation and keep her from moving. In some settings, the beds will move and in others the machine will move. That way, the beams will be more likely to hit the target exactly. The machines that move will be controlled in another room next to the patient's room. They are adjusted by the radiation therapist according to the patient's tumor location, marked by the tattoo.

The patient cannot smell or feel the radiation. She will know when it starts and finishes by the click of the machine. The treatment is painless and usually takes between 5-30 minutes. Then, she will be wheeled into a recovery room. The start and finish times will be noted by the radiation team, as well as the doses and locations. The radiation therapist will record the dosage information in the patient's medical file.

What This Procedure Means for You

As the patient is receiving treatment, you will be in a separate room. The activity involved to deliver the treatment may take considerably longer than 30 minutes, especially if there is extra care that needs to be given to her. This may take a while, but you won't want to rush this.

Remember that radiation can be extremely harmful if received in uncontrolled doses. If the radiation team asks you to wait an extra long time or gives you careful instructions about interacting with the patient after you see her, *do as instructed.* You need to keep yourself mentally and physically healthy. When it is safe for you to see her, they will notify you. Over the next 25-30 visits, you can keep yourself sane by using some of the strategies of Winning the Waiting Game.

Chemotherapy

"He met these two other patients in the infusion room, and now it's like Friday Night Poker," says Tilda, 70. "Only it's Tuesday at 10 a.m. and they only have three players. But, the doctor lets them have that deck of cards and some plastic chips and they pass the time together while getting chemo. I wonder if he looks a little forward to it."

What is Happening to the Patient

Chemotherapy, or chemo, can be given in a variety of settings: at home, in the doctor's office, in a clinic, hospital, outpatient facility, or hospital. Typically, chemotherapy is infused, which means it is given INTRAVENOUSLY (by IV) in a special infusion room at an ONCOLOGY office or in a hospital room. A patient may be in a room with several other patients or he may be in a room by himself. Usually, he will have BLOOD COUNTS taken before the treatment, so that the oncologist will be able to measure the effect of the therapy.

The oncology nurse will prepare the IV with the chemo agents. The patient is usually in bed or a reclining chair with a television at his disposal. He will normally receive the medicine through an IV in the arm or PORTACATH. Like other medicines given by IV, chemo can be felt as it circulates through the body. Depending on the PROTOCOL, it can take a short time or several hours. When the medicine is finished, he will be encouraged to rest. After this, the patient can usually return home. With later appointments, blood counts will again be taken, and the results will be compared with his initial counts. If the counts are low, he may be given more blood or blood products to keep up adequate blood counts.

If the patient takes chemo orally (by pill) at home, there are guidelines how and when to take it. There will be no IV involved with these doses. Be sure he follows the instructions on the label, especially in terms of what foods or beverages are to be consumed with each dose.

What This Procedure Means for You

Depending on the setting, you may be able to accompany the patient as he is getting the chemo. Caregivers talk about holding the patient's hand while he takes the pill or while the nurse prepares the treatment. But you may need to sit in another room, outside the infusion room, while the patient receives the chemotherapy.

Some oncology nurses say that patients enjoy being in a group setting in the infusion room. Like Tilda's husband in the quote above, they may feel like they are not alone. Each patient is different, though. As the weeks progress, you will be able to estimate when it's important for you to be with the patient and how long the appointments will be. There's a prime opportunity to use the strategies of Winning the Waiting Game.

Managing Relationships with Medical Professionals

Throughout this journey, the patient's medical professionals have guided you. As you continue the relationships with them, you will experience the importance of being an effective advocate for the patient while understanding and carrying out their recommendations for care. When wrapping up the treatment visit to take the patient home, you will need to get some information from them about the outpatient care needs – those that will be handled at home by you.

Many doctors will give you printed instructions to address outpatient care needs. Read them. The tips they give you will make life back at home easier. If they don't provide instructions, ask for their assistance to put together a short list of expected outcomes. Talk to them about what is likely to happen and what to do about it if it does. The list that results from the discussion may look something like this:

IF: Patient has discomfort at the INCISION SITE.

THEN: Call the physician's assistance or nurse practitioner for instructions.

IF: Patient has trouble sleeping.

THEN: Give the patient the prescription sleep aid according to the prescribed dose. Or, try another approach which may suit the patient's situation.

You probably won't need a first aid certification to facilitate minor patient care, but you will need to know what to do if symptoms become impossible to manage. By going over several expected outcomes with the healthcare providers, you should be able to determine which ones you could handle on your own and which ones you can't.

If you think it will be hard for you to meet some of his needs with your current abilities, ask about the possibility of using volunteers or a home health nurse. Often, insurance covers additional professional assistance immediately after treatment. Many hospitals also have access to local volunteers. Though they may be untrained, they will usually help for free and are wonderful assets.

What Do I Say? Questions for the Medical Professionals at Patient Discharge

Bringing the patient home after treatment can be emotional. If you're having trouble forming the questions to ask the medical professionals then, here are some ideas:

- What are the prescriptions and are there special diet considerations?

- How do I care for special aids, such as tubes or drains?

- Are there special considerations when dressing or moving the patient? What would you recommend in terms of activity, showering, exercising, or driving?

- What is considered an emergency? Who do we call with questions, during or after business hours?

- When should we come in for a check-up?

Before you leave the treatment facility, be sure you have the information you need. Then you'll be ready to go home and continue care according to your Care Plan.

Heading Home From Treatment

"We learned Italian in the car," says Maria, 68. "We decided we wanted to visit our relatives in Italy after Rich's treatment was done. So we called the trip our 'graduation present' and made a goal to enjoy the time to and from each treatment."

After a treatment, you'll have another opportunity to help the patient with mobility, as he may be even weaker and more fatigued than before treatment. Don't be surprised if you're tired, too. Go slowly when moving him. Follow the procedures mentioned earlier to get him into and out of the car comfortably without hurting yourself. The patient will likely want to rest, but he may also want to talk. If so, let him decide how much and about what. The important things to keep in mind are that this particular treatment is done and you are both one step closer to beating the cancer.

If you pass a pharmacy on the way home, consider stopping to fill prescriptions or other medical supplies. This way, you'll have what you need to carry out the Care Plan at home and you'll save yourself another trip.

Taking Care of Yourself

*"I feel like everyone wants a piece of me," says Tammy, 38.
"I'm responsible for my kids, my husband, my work, the dog,
and now my mom. I'm exhausted. I can't think. I feel like I'm
on the edge of an emotional cliff. When did I give up my own
life?"*

Caring for a patient who is going through treatment is very challenging
for the caregiver and the process can be very draining. Continuing to
care for someone during a treatment may be doubly difficult if you, a
primary caregiver, are *exhausted.* You may see yourself like Tammy
in the quote above – your Personal Enemy #1 is not the patient's
cancer right now. It's COMPASSION FATIGUE.

Most caregivers are so unaware of this that they don't even recognize
the name. Compassion fatigue attacks those who care for one or more
people besides themselves. It is the mental, physical and emotional
toll that stress and trauma take. You may know it as burnout or
feeling wired and tired. It's easy to forget about yourself and fall into
this unhealthy trap.

Don't let yourself turn into the second patient. Give yourself
permission to be healthy in mind, body, and spirit, even when the
patient is not. Pay attention to your body's symptoms of exhaustion
and problems with attention or coordination. If you are able to keep
yourself strong, you will be more likely to give good care, make good
decisions, and have energy when the patient does not. You've made
it this far – You can do it!

How Can I Help Myself? Avoiding Compassion Fatigue

Be easy on yourself. Being responsible for someone's survival is
new territory. Expect to make some mistakes. You are not an expert
now, but you can and you will learn. Ask questions. Talk to case
managers, social workers, and other counselors in the hospital or at
the doctor's office.

Don't judge yourself – what comes out of your mouth could seem strange to others, but you're just not thinking straight. Instead, encourage yourself every day. You are both competent and confident.

Visualizing your life when the patient is well can be rejuvenating. Start a plan of escape. Think about what you might do when the caregiving experience is over. She will not be sick forever. Allow it to be your goal and your daydream when you are in pain, grieving, or fatigued.

Do something just for you. Even when money is tight and time is nonexistent, take 10 minutes to eat an ice cream bar, buy flowers for yourself, open a paperback, use a new toothbrush, scatter some seeds, play the lottery. Search out a quiet place. Go there to be uninterrupted, even if only for a few minutes.

When Others Ask "How Can I Help?" *20 Ideas to Let Them*

The best way to avoid compassion fatigue is by delegating to others. When people want to help, give them this list. Have them:

1. Baby sit. Take the kids or the patient to an amusement park.

2. Rent a movie and watch it with the patient. Bring popcorn or pizza.

3. Drive. Take the children to destinations, pick up prescriptions, drive the patient to doctors, transport out-of-town guests, or deliver groceries.

4. Listen without judging.

5. Learn a new skill with the patient. Sign up for classes together.

6. Spend time with the patient to see what energy level he has. Start some other project to ease his mind or distract him, helping him contribute even in his weakened state. Can he hull strawberries or fold clothing or spread mulch?

7. Bring the patient a few books, magazines, or music from the library.

8. Provide extra rooms or meals for out-of-town guests.

9. Bring a child to visit the patient when he is up to it. Coloring, playing games, and storytelling are all wonderful gifts from children.

10. Plan something fun. Go to a comedy club or plan a joke fest dinner wherever you can. Just bring your favorite riddle or funny story.

11. Use the internet to take a virtual tour of a zoo or museum.

12. Help with seasonal needs – put on snow tires, plow, salt, cover plants, fertilize, take down storm windows and put up screens, clean the gutters, rake leaves.

13. Decorate for the holidays. Put up decorations or take them down. Celebrate together as much as possible.

14. Do some special holiday cooking and baking.

15. Organize a community event to make cards, raise funds, or just inspire the patient and caregiver.

16. Pull out the home movies.

17. Create a poem or song and perform it for the patient.

18. Offer a specialty to the patient with love, no matter what it is – cooking, singing, knitting, scrapbook-making, financial planning, or cutting hair.

19. Do something anonymously in her name. Perhaps you could donate to a favorite cause, dedicate a religious service.

20. Start a prayer or meditation list at a place of worship.

Wrapping Up

You are doing something really wonderful by helping the patient through treatment.

It's easy to feel that you're losing control in a situation that seems ever-changing. No two illnesses or patients are alike. Though you may have the best Care Team, the course of the illness may not be predictable.

To keep your sanity and your health during the patient's treatment, remember:

- You can win the Waiting Game by making the time productive for you. That can mean resting, doing something for the patient, or doing something for yourself.

- You should understand the patient's needs before leaving the care facility.

- Give yourself loving care to avoid compassion fatigue. Taking care of yourself will enable you to provide the patient the level of care you strive for.

- You can involve others in the patient's care to give yourself a well-earned break.

Look how much you've learned! You've made it through the first part of treatment with the patient. The next chapter will tackle how you will care for the patient at home between treatments.

Chapter 7: Providing Care at Home Between Treatments

"My wife's recovery from surgery was difficult and she had a lot of ongoing problems," says Bill, 50. "When it came time for her to go home, we were very anxious about knowing what was usual versus what was serious that the doctors needed to know about. After all, everything was serious to us. Thankfully, the surgeon, his physician assistant, and his nurse practitioner continued to answer our questions and got us through the most difficult period – the first couple of weeks home from the hospital."

When the patient meets the criteria to go home after a procedure, it's completely normal to be worried. While the medical professionals are confident about releasing the patient to your care, you may not be confident in yourself. Have faith! They are confident that the patient is stable and that you can address outcomes that surface. We have faith in you too.

Remember the Care Plan we talked about a few chapters ago? If you were able to put one together, now's the time to pull it out and use it. If you weren't, don't worry. In this chapter, we'll help you to:

- Anticipate Common Outcomes to Traditional Treatments

- Manage His Pain (and Other Symptoms) Without Having Some of Your Own

- Master Daily Challenges – Part I

- Tame "The Impossible Patient"

- Lasso Runaway Stress

- Take Care of Yourself.

The more prepared to you, the easier it will be to deal with the impacts of the disease – on the patient and on *you*. Caregiving at home can be the most difficult part of caregiving and it *will* take a toll on you. To avoid major negative impacts, you'll need to act with Rule #1 in mind: You must maintain an even balance between the patient's concerns and your personal concerns. This applies to the whole caregiving process. Even when you're caring for the patient at home, it is OK to watch out for yourself. At the end of this chapter, like the others, are suggestions on taking care of yourself. It merits repeating to tell you to take advantage of them when you can. It may be hard to tend to the patient at home and to also take care of yourself, but read on. We're going to do it the best way we know how.

Using Your Care Plan

Whether or not you put together a formal Care Plan, you've made decisions about professionals, heathcare facilities, and treatments. Now you're seeing some of those decisions turn into action as the procedure takes place, and you can evaluate how your plans came out. You've probably also thought about how the patient would be cared for at home after treatment. Now you'll have a chance to put those thoughts into action.

Reactions to treatments are highly individual. No one experiences all forms of expected outcomes or SIDE EFFECTS. You will not know in advance how the outcomes or side effects will surface or how they will affect your lifestyle. You will find yourself reacting to them when the patient starts experiencing them.

However, you can take some precautions by reading the materials from the doctor and scheduling a home healthcare nurse or volunteer if you need one. You can also:

- Assemble a very basic home health kit. You may already have things at home for handling cuts, infections, fever, headaches, or minor pains.

- Understand the intent of prescription medication. Fill the prescriptions and have the patient take them as they are prescribed. Sometimes this means *before* symptoms are present.

- Get familiar with dosage instructions, timing, and specific handling instructions for each medicine. If it is taken by another route than by mouth, ask the nurse to demonstrate how to give the medicine before you try to give it on your own.

The next table gives you a summary of common outcomes of procedures to give you a starting point on what to expect. Don't worry – Assistance is coming: The sections that follow will help you and the patient manage them. Then, there are ideas for mastering the daily challenges associated with them. We will get through it all.

Anticipating Common Treatment Outcomes

Following Surgery		
• Abdominal bloating and mild cramping • Constipation from pain medicines • Decreased mental sharpness from anesthesia • Decreased mobility or movement	• Discomfort at incision site • Disturbed sleep/wake cycles • Energy loss/fatigue • Blood clotting (DEEP VEIN THROMBOSIS)	• Nausea and vomiting • Scar tissue formation • Swelling at the site (LYMPHEDEMA) • Weight loss, limited appetite, decreased food and fluid intake
Following Radiation		
• Decreased mobility or movement • Diarrhea, stomach aches and cramps (lower abdomen) • Difficulty swallowing (head, neck, chest, lung, or esophagus) • Energy loss, fatigue	• Hair loss in radiated area • Impact to hearing (head, neck, upper-chest) • Limited appetite, weight loss, decreased food and fluid intake • Mouth sores, loss of salivary function	• Nausea, vomiting and bloating (upper abdomen) • Skin changes or scarring • Swelling at the site or lymphedema • Voice impairment (head, neck, upper-chest)
Following Chemotherapy		
• ANEMIA, low platelet and white blood cell counts, increased risk of infection • Decreased mental sharpness, memory loss (called CHEMO BRAIN) • Diarrhea • Nausea and vomiting	• Difficulty breathing • Energy loss, fatigue • Hair loss • Numbness or tingling in fingers and toes (NEUROPATHY)	• Impotence • Low appetite, weight loss • Mouth sores • Slow growth of skin and nails, discoloration

Handling Troubling Treatment Outcomes

While many of the treatment outcomes can be worrisome, these are generally the most troubling: pain, fatigue, problems with elimination of waste, and ALOPECIA (hair loss).

We'll take a look at these first.

Managing His Pain without Having Some of Your Own

"We were trying to figure out where the pain came from and what made it better or worse," says Trudy, 55. "Don was worried about taking the opiates – he didn't want to be out of control or become an addict. I think 'manliness' had something to do with it too – him feeling like he should be able to take it and not show his 'weakness' in front of the kids or his friends. The pain was, by far, our biggest and scariest concern."

Pain is an individual sensation of discomfort. It may be mild or severe, constant or intermittent. If left untreated, pain can affect mood, energy levels, concentration, and even romantic life. In short, it can reduce the overall quality of life.

What exactly causes pain? In cancer patients, pain may surface because a TUMOR has invaded bones, nerves, or body organs, causing sensitivity or damage to the structure. It can accompany testing. Or, it may surface in treatment recovery because of lack of activity (causing cramping or bedsores) or reactivation of joints or muscles that haven't been used in a while.

If the patient is in pain and his regular, over-the-counter medicines aren't working, *get help.* Not all health professionals are specialists in pain management, but most have general training and they can give you several options. When deciding on the best approach for managing or eliminating pain, doctors and their staff members will ask questions to find the cause of pain and to understand its characteristics. For this reason, you and he must be able to evaluate the pain and to talk about it.

What Do I Say? Questions for Describing the Pain

Pain can be difficult to describe. You can begin by having the patient point out exactly where it hurts. Then guide him as he describes it, with questions like these:

- When did it start and when does it happen? Is it every once in a while or continuously?

- What does it feel like (aching, burning, sharpness, stabbing, throbbing)?

- How bad is the pain on a scale of 0-10? Think of 0 as being no pain and 10 as being "the worst pain you've ever had" or pain that is "paralyzing."

- Has the pain changed or moved? What makes it better or worse?

- Do you have other symptoms with the pain, like sweating or nausea?

Write down or memorize his answers, so that you'll be able to reiterate them to the medical professional. If you have an idea of what might be causing the pain, write that down as well. It may prove to be valuable in finding the pain's source and its solution.

How Can I Help? Managing the Pain

People in pain can be mean-spirited, angry, and even violent. It can be difficult to control someone else's pain and to watch someone suffer. If the patient is in pain, you should manage it by putting together a plan with your healthcare providers.

Cancer pain is traditionally treated with medicine. Pain medicine is given in various forms, usually by mouth (orally), through injection or IV, applied to the skin (transdermally), around the spine (epidurally), or as a suppository (rectally). Sometimes, the patient is given a pain pump or Patient Controlled Analgesia (PCA). This is an IV with a button that he can press to release pain medicine into the bloodstream. This way, he can receive the medication according to his needs. The overall dose is regulated, however, to avoid possible overdose or addiction.

No matter how the medicine is given, the patient needs to be aware that:

- Most pain medicine is prescribed to be taken as needed. You will know that because PRN or PRO RE NATA may appear on the prescription. Take this type of medication when the pain is mild so the medicine can work as the pain increases in intensity.

- If pain medication is prescribed on a regular schedule, do not skip doses. That may result in breakthrough pain, which requires rescue doses of other pain medications. These rescue doses often take an hour or more before they are effective and therefore the patient would be in pain during that time.

- If a medication does not seem to be working, ask the medical professionals to find another that does.

For persistent pain, pain medicine may not be enough. Pain Management specialists may consider other options such as surgery, hormone therapy, and radiation therapy, depending on the situation. In addition, there are multiple complementary therapies that have shown varying degrees of success in managing pain. The complementary therapies included in the next section are more commonly accepted by traditional medicine practitioners for addressing pain of various forms.

Using Complementary Therapies for Pain Management

Patients and their caregivers are often willing to try a variety of complementary therapies to combat severe or repetitive effects from the treatment, the medication, or the illness itself. Some of these techniques are described here. Be aware that there are risks based on the individual's overall health and treatment history. When trying these, use caution. This information is included to potentially help both you and the patient, not to contradict what your medical professionals have outlined for the patient.

- Acupressure – Pressure points on the body are pressed and massaged to facilitate healing, flexibility, and balance. The best way to experience this is through an experienced practitioner.

- Acupuncture – Pins are inserted into special points on the skin to trigger and internal change in energy flow for pain relief. Use a certified professional for this technique.

- Hypnotherapy – Specialists believe that the mind-body connection can help to identify pain in the body and move through it with relaxation and tension release, using both self-hypnotherapy and therapy with a qualified hypnotist. However, there is some question about the use of hypnotherapy for those with a history of mental illness, so do not approach this therapy without consulting a qualified hypnotist and the patient's medical professional.

- Massage – In many cultures, touch plays an important part in healing by easing muscle tension. A word of caution: Avoid working at or around areas that are injured, operated upon, currently irradiated, or used for IVs and PORTACATHS. Massage is intended to promote healing, not to incur damage or soreness. Hiring a professional is one option and self-massage is another. If you're interested in learning how to do this, several books and pamphlets offer suggestions and instructions.

- Meditation – Meditation involves clearing the mind to help the body focus on healing. Book stores and music stores carry meditation CDs, tapes, or DVDs that can help you get started.

- Prayer – Spirituality is a very private matter, often hinging on your cultural background. Some patients find that direct communication with their higher power gives them a sense of relief or release. Prayer can be silent or verbal, spoken or sung, group or individual. If you're interested in praying, some people say you can't do it wrong – it's as easy as thinking or talking.

- Visualization – Do you remember daydreaming as a child? Do you remember a time recently where you could almost see how you want things to be? Some adults call this 'wishful thinking' but it's also visualization. Visualization can help identify what you really want and how it could happen for you. You can also imagine something beautiful or peaceful, like fireflies or hummingbirds.

- Reflexology – Some consider this a type of massage, where other parts of the body (internal and external) are indirectly massaged via the feet. A foot map has been established, linking different parts of the body to different parts of the feet. The idea behind this is that problem areas can be approached for healing without direct contact with that part of the body.

Because these are complementary therapies, they may be used in combination with medication and other pain management procedures. Use what works best for the patient and for you.

Fighting Fatigue

"We both wonder 'Will I ever get my energy back?'" says Maggie, 48. "We laugh but then realize it's sad that neither one of us is at 100%. And I'm not even sick."

We all get tired. But fatigue is extreme, prolonged weariness and total lack of energy. People recognize fatigue when they are having difficulty performing simple tasks such as taking a shower, climbing stairs, or even concentrating. This challenge affects both patients and caregivers.

What exactly causes fatigue? Fatigue can be caused by changes to the nervous system, or physical and emotional stresses. It can also be caused by dehydration or not eating/poor nutrition, a lack of exercise, or the effects of medications. Not getting enough sleep can be a factor as well, especially when a patient needs extra sleep and energy to heal from treatment or infection.

Fatigue can be accompanied by shortness of breath, tingling or burning feelings in arms or legs, or loss of balance. Unfortunately, this sometimes discourages patients from trying to exercise or engage in physical activity, which are two great ways to fight fatigue.

How Can I Help? Conserving Energy and Rebuilding Strength

Most cancer patients and many caregivers experience fatigue at some point during the course of the disease. These ideas will help both of you to fight it:

- Arrange your routine based on flows in your energy levels. That is, work while you're energized and rest when you're not. If certain things have to be done at a certain time, ask for some assistance.

- Choose one goal for the day, hour, or week. Put the energy you have into accomplishing that one priority. Forgive yourself for not being able to do any other tasks during that time.

- Get plenty of rest. If you need sleep medication, ask for it.

- Keep snacks on hand. Eat small meals frequently. Consider baby food as an alternative if the patient is having trouble eating.

- Drink nutritional supplements or drinks.

- If the idea of exercising is intimidating to either you or the patient, start by wiggling the toes or bending and straightening the knees. Try walking a little. Then walk a little more.

- Work with the physical therapy staff or a personal trainer to identify range of motion exercises to help the patient overcome trouble with moving.

- If you have the stamina, search out fitness classes or weight training programs.

- If you're not having trouble moving but you need to increase your endurance, buy or borrow some supplies. Hand weights, rubber balls, exercise cables, or an exercise bike can help slowly build strength and coordination with little chance of injury.

Remember that fighting fatigue is challenging. You may both need encouragement for every step you take, so be generous with your support and your praise.

Dealing with Waste Elimination

"No one likes to talk about this kind of thing," says Leila, 67. "In my day, you just didn't mention it if you had trouble in the bathroom. But it seems like we have to talk about it with our doctors to get my husband some relief. Your pride, along with many other things, goes down the drain."

Most people take the regular elimination of waste from the body for granted. But when there are problems with this, it can be extremely uncomfortable and in severe cases, serious. It's also not that comfortable to talk about, so many people avoid telling their medical professionals about the problems, when they could have been corrected with little effort.

Some of the common situations are put in a chart that follows. Like many of the other situations in this chapter, these will often reverse themselves to regular functioning with time. If they persist, there may be medical concerns that are causing or adding to these problems. Be clear on who to contact: the last thing you'll want to do is fumble around for a number or a name in the phone book when you need it. Contact the medical professional who is in charge of the patient's specific treatment: the oncologist (CHEMOTHERAPY), the radiation oncologist (radiation), or the surgical oncologist/surgeon (surgery). Have that number and the number of a backup close at hand.

Handling Challenges With Eliminating Waste

Situation	How Can I Help?
Diarrhea	• Suggest that he stay near to a restroom. Keep extra toilet paper or tissues close by. • Try medicated wipes to soothe the sore rear end. Topical or local pain medicines can decrease discomfort as well. • Some doctors recommend a clear liquid diet of water, broth, juice, plain gelatin, weak tea, and sports drinks. • Specific medications are designed to stop this.
Constipation	• Under advisement of the healthcare team, reduce narcotic pain medication. • Help him stay hydrated with plenty of liquids such as water, broth, sports drinks, and juice (especially prune juice). • Encourage him to eat fruits and vegetables. • Ask your doctor if bulking products, stool softeners, and laxatives will help. • Promote regular exercise.
Cramping	• Stretch with the patient if the cramping is in places other than the abdomen. Try anti-spasmodic medicines for abdominal cramping.
Flatulence	• Ask him to avoid eating gas-forming foods like beans. • Consider gas relief products that are available over the counter.

Situation	How Can I Help?
Bladder and Urinary Tract Infections	• Make sure that the patient has an adequate intake of fluids to release urine regularly. Ask the doctor what adequate will mean for you in terms of cups or glasses. • Consider having him drink cranberry juice to help the body heal the infection.
Incontinence	• Encourage the patient to do Kegel exercises to strengthen muscles controlling this. In women, these muscles are in the inner lining of the vaginal walls. In men, these muscles are at the base of the pelvis. Contraction and release of the muscles controls the flow or urine.

Anticipating Alopecia

*"Hair always grows back, at least from what I've seen,"
says Candie, 40. "As a salon owner, I have worked on a
number of cancer patients. It may come back brown when
it was previously grey or curly where it was straight before.
But it always grows back. That's why I can assure my dad it
will come back for him, too."*

Alopecia is the medical term for the thinning and loss of hair. Alopecia
from some cancer treatments occurs not only on a person's head, but
all over the body including legs, underarm, and pubic hair. Hair is
present on most parts of people's bodies. Hair adds color, warmth,
and dimension to our bodies, and without it we feel naked. Many
people are concerned with hair loss, thinking that it is a certainty
that they will lose their hair with chemotherapy. But not all drugs or
combination of drugs cause it.

Hair loss happens because certain chemotherapy does not distinguish
between types of quickly-reproducing cells: it affects hair follicles
and other healthy cells when attacking the CANCER CELLS. New hair
does not grow for a short time, but the existing hair will continue

to move out of the scalp or other skin as though it had new growth behind it. Consequently, without the anchor of new hair growth, the existing hair will detach from its follicle. The patient may experience clumps falling out in his hands or see the result on a pillow or in the shower. Hair loss can be quite traumatic, especially on those with longer hair, where the amount of detached hair is much more noticeable.

If it is going to happen, hair doesn't start falling out until two to three weeks after treatment begins. It may fall out gradually, in clumps, or even all at once. But it will likely grow back about two to three weeks after the patient finishes chemo.

How Can I Help? When the Patient is Losing Hair

Caregivers recommend talking to the patient's hairstylist or barber to anticipate possible effects to the scalp and hair after chemotherapy. You may be surprised at the suggestions they have about frequency of trimmings, what products to use for sensitive scalps, and how to fit and style wigs. They may even offer to shop with the patient for wigs, turbans, or hats. There are styles available for both women and men, like press boy caps, baseball hats, or fishing hats. While you're shopping, you may also want to buy the patient a new razor and great shaving cream to remind them that the hair will grow back. It will help them look forward to this sign of healing.

Here are some other tips:

Have a portable vacuum cleaner within reach to collect the hair that is lost in bed, in the car, or in the bathroom. Hair is easier to collect when it is dry. If possible, use soft fabric pillowcases, like satin or flannel, for the patient to sleep on. Apply moisturizer often to the scalp and other sensitive areas. Some may also want to brush on eyebrows if the loss is noticeable. In general, pay attention to the patient's attitude about the hair loss and adjust to it. Remind the patient that the hair loss is almost always temporary.

Managing Other Expected Outcomes

It's difficult to name every possible outcome, so we'll cover just five more. Take another deep breath. If and when these things happen, you can help.

Handling Common Outcomes

Situation	How Can I Help?
Nausea and Vomiting	• Keep buckets and towels at ready access at home and in the car. • Ask about medications called anti-emedic drugs to reduce nausea and vomiting that are often prescribed for the patient to take before nausea starts. • Prepare soft, bland foods such as animal crackers, rice, mashed potatoes, or oatmeal. Prepare plenty of liquids too, like soup, juice, or non-carbonated drinks. Feed the patient when he can eat. • Position the patient to sit upright after eating. • Suggest smaller, more frequent meals. • Ventilate food areas. Keep him away from strong odors.
Blood clotting difficulties, such as bleeding gums or nose. Prolonged bleeding or excessive bruising could follow a minor trauma.	• Avoid aspirin or other medicines that may thin the blood. • Keep dark towels, which won't stain, around to clean up blood. • Ask the patient's medical professionals about these options: replacing or enhancing his production of blood-clotting components or receiving additional blood and blood products.

Situation	How Can I Help?
Skin and nail changes, including dryness, sunburns, irritation, pigment changes, itching.	• Pamper the skin with creams, lotions, and mild soaps that are moisturizing. Be sure to get approval from the medical professional first. • Avoid perfume, adhesive tapes, hot or cold packs. • Use soft sponges and lukewarm water to bathe area. Add oatmeal, mild bath salts, or cornstarch to the water. • Use an electric shaver if he must shave. • Stay out of the pool and the sunlight.
Fluid Retention	• Hormones, such as prednisone, cause fluid to be retained. Consider having these levels adjusted or asking the doctor to prescribe diuretics to release the fluid. • Avoid feeding the patient high-sodium foods like ham or potato chips.
Numbness	• There may be multiple causes for this. Talk to the doctor to determine the underlying cause and treat it appropriately.
Change in Vision	• Do not rush out to get a new set of contacts or glasses. Ask about the permanency of the change and make adjustments accordingly.

Keep in mind that many of these outcomes and side effects reverse themselves when a patient finishes treatment. They will, however, affect daily living during treatment. The next few sections will give you ideas to get through these challenges.

Mastering Daily Challenges – Part I

Get ready, because your day-to-day routine is about to change. During treatment, there's a possibility, even a probability, that the patient will need assistance with many things he could previously do by himself. Suddenly, regular activity may seem like tasks for Hercules instead of him. Without you, activities like eating, dressing, and moving may be difficult, if not out of the question.

You want to provide the best patient care with the least impact to your routine. So you'll need to have an idea of what is likely to happen and what to do when it does – which includes getting help if you need it. Let's take a look at some daily activities and the challenges that may accompany them. You'll find that they will be easier to master when you can anticipate them. Involve the other members of your Care Team and take advantage of the services you've discovered in creating your Care Plan to lighten this caregiving load. They are there to help you.

Managing Meals and Changing Nutritional Needs

"We had so much food in the house," said Jim, 44, caring for his wife with breast cancer. "I think my friends thought I would starve because Mary wasn't cooking. She wasn't eating either – so sick and so tired from the chemotherapy.

"She also had these awful mouth sores. I thought surely she would eat some of the food they brought. At least the desserts. Normally, she has a bit of a sweet tooth. But the desserts just sat there. She tried once or twice to eat and just threw everything up. Then her mouth hurt twice as much.

"Finally, someone suggested frozen juices and desserts. These were great because they iced down her mouth sores and didn't upset her stomach. She ate quite a few of those. I think she didn't mind them being sweet, either."

Cancer treatment often brings issues with eating such as loss of appetite, weight loss, and new food sensitivities. These obstacles have physical and emotional effects. Facing them can be extra tough because patients usually eat three or more times per day. You'll need to balance when the patient wants to eat against changing nutritional needs and physical capabilities. While the medical professionals may be encouraged by treatment results, you and the patient may feel discouraged by unexpected side effects. Thankfully, many of these obstacles are short-term: as patients heal, meal times usually go back to normal routines.

In the meantime, try to save her favorite foods until her treatments are over. They usually taste better then. Buy foods that you can easily prepare and eat. When you have some time to cook, cook larger quantities and freeze leftovers for a later meal. You could try having one special meal each week (eaten out, cooked by a friend, or as a picnic). Make it fun – select a theme, make decorations, try a new recipe. As a change of pace, it will give you and the patient something to look forward to.

With treatments like chemotherapy, the patient's immune system may be compromised. Cancer is not contagious but other diseases are. During food preparation and cooking, watch for contamination, fungus, and mold, such as foods or liquids with strange smells or coloration. Be wary, because bacteria can spread through the air, insects, food, tables, countertops, non-sterile clothing, or equipment.

When you're planning a meal, you may also have to consider a few other obstacles besides those that are food-related. Some common obstacles and ways to approach them appear in the next chart. Again, if any of these conditions becomes severe, call your medical professional.

Handling Challenges With Meals and Nutrition

Situation	How Can I Help?
Bedridden	• Learn how to gently move the patient and help him eat while sitting up. Clean up any food spilled on him and in the bed.
Cannot feed himself	• Do your best to feed the patient through the mouth with small bites and soft foods. Talk to the medical professional about tube-feeding or IV nutrition, if appropriate. Over the long-term, find a physical therapist to help him regain the physical ability to feed himself. There are devices to help eat and drink, like angled spoons and two-handled cups.

Situation	How Can I Help?
Has feeding tubes, liquid feeding, or gastric drainage bags for surgery patients	• Many people have no experience with these items, which can be frustrating to manage without training. The visiting nurse will teach you how to give meals, how to take care of the equipment, and how to maintain good hygiene.
Experiences pain while eating or swallowing. Patient may have throat sores, dry mouth/salivation problems, mouth sores, thrush, or tooth decay.	• Certain types of mouthwash can be prescribed to manage pain or to cure mouth sores. The patient may also want to try baking soda and warm water (instead of mouthwash with alcohol) to rinse the mouth. • If she wants to brush, try children's toothpaste on a cotton swab, instead of a toothbrush. • Keep her mouth moist with ice chips, sugarless gum, or candy. • Serve nutritional drinks and soft foods, like fruit smoothies, milkshakes, applesauce, eggs, rice, pasta, cottage cheese, macaroni and cheese, pudding, oatmeal or hot soft cereals, yogurt, or cream soups. Use the food processor or blender to soften foods. • Avoid serving very hot or spicy foods, crackers, nuts, raw vegetables, chips, or other food that may hurt when eating. • For tea drinkers, try peppermint or chamomile tea.
Has no appetite or has a different eating schedule than the caregiver.	• Let the patient eat at her own pace, and at her own times, when possible. Eating only a couple of bites is better than not eating at all. • Consider helping her eat on a schedule, as with medication doses. Make flavorful food in small quantities at specific times. Decide whether you want to follow the dietary restrictions and schedule yourself. • Ask the oncologist about medicines that are appetite stimulators. • Give the patient plenty of water.

Moving, Washing, and Dressing the Patient

"Getting around was pretty easy, even during the treatment,"
says Walt, 70, whose wife has been diagnosed with uterine
cancer. "We just needed a few instructions, a little practice,
and the help of some medical equipment."

When the patient can generally move by herself, you may not need to be concerned with how she walks, bathes, or dresses. However, if the patient is challenged with fatigue, muscle loss, nausea, or pain, all of these things can be difficult for her. Often, you'll find that she'll be weakened from treatment or from the cancer itself. The good news is that the obstacles in moving, washing, and dressing the patient can be overcome easily after they are identified. In fact, you've probably already had some success just getting the patient to treatment.

Here are some hints: Helping someone to walk up and down stairs requires a different technique than helping someone bathe. To move the patient, get training from the nursing or physical therapy staffs on techniques and safety. Make sure the move makes sense to you. Do you have to do it? Are you capable of doing it alone? If not, can someone help?

Don't attempt a move if you're not comfortable with it – and that includes washing and dressing the patient. If you must move the patient alone, check the floors for items that may cause tripping or slipping like clothes on the floor or water. It can be very dangerous to try to move a patient in a wet and slippery situation. Move slowly to avoid cuts, bruises, and broken bones. If that happens, take the patient (or yourself) in for medical care.

Hygiene is especially important during treatment, when the immune system may be compromised and the risk of infection may be higher. So whether the patient washes on her own or with your help, it's critical that she stays as clean as possible.

When the patient can generally wash by herself, let her. If she needs help, help her gently. You may have to evaluate that on your own because some patients do not ask for it.

Asking for assistance with washing and dressing is considered by many to be the height of dependency. Sometimes there is a simple fix, like placing a small chair in the shower so that she can sit as she washes. Other times, cleaning the patient may be more involved.

Sponge baths, when the patient is gently cleaned in bed with soap, water, sponges, and washcloths, may be required if she has difficulty leaving the bed. If necessary, ask the nursing staff for advice on when to wash, locations to target or avoid, and approaches to wash someone who is lying down.

When the patient can generally dress herself, the challenge is to choose clothing that she'll likely need after her treatment. Depending on the treatment type, the patient's clothing needs will vary. Here are some guidelines to tell her.

- Stay away from tight clothing. Wear loose garments that can be put on over the head and fastened with snaps or elastic.

- With skin sensitivities, wear softer fabrics and styles that do not brush against the affected area. The patient may want to wear gloves, long sleeves, or long pants to prevent scratches, burns, or cuts. When carrying a purse, have her use hand straps instead of shoulder straps.

- After chemotherapy, wear hats or scarves to protect the head from sunburn or cold weather if there is hair loss.

- With swelling (LYMPHEDEMA), dress the affected limb with compression garments to minimize swelling.

- With bandaged incisions, choose styles that protect the affected areas.

- To hide scars, find clothing that is long enough to cover the scar.

- To accommodate drains, appliances, or prosthetics, select comfortable garments that move with the device, like unfitted tops or pants with elastic waists.

- For women who have recently had breast surgery, try special bras constructed of cotton and other soft fabrics without metal fastenings, such as exercise/jog bras. Some are fitted with breast forms.

If the patient has limited mobility, ask the nursing staff for some training on how to gently guide her into and out of clothing. The dressing process will vary with treatment type, as well as the patient's overall agility and desire to change clothing. Keep in mind that most of these adjustments are short-term and they can help prepare you for the long-term changes.

A Few Words on Disposing of Medical and Bodily Waste

Personal healthcare items, such as unused medications, syringes, or needles that are intended for the patient need to be disposed of properly. It is important that no other adults, children, or pets find them. Misuse of them could cause serious problems including death. Many nurses recommend putting needles and syringes inside a sturdy, colored plastic container (like an empty laundry detergent bottle) before throwing them in the trash.

Unused medication should not be flushed down the toilet. Changing the form of medicine may help to keep it out of the wrong hands or mouths. Add water to pills and other solid medication in their containers to dissolve them. Add sand, flour, or kitty litter to liquid medicines to solidify them.

You may also have concerns about disposing bodily waste. The waste can take several forms, including blood, urine, vomit, and feces. Encountering waste is often unpleasant and the odor can be nauseating to you as well.

If you come across bodily waste from the patient, act quickly. Make her comfortable first and then start cleaning. Most waste can be picked up with a towel. Do not use your hands. Use dark colored towels to mop waste up, because they will be less likely to stain. Feces and larger food particles from vomit can be disposed of down the toilet. Wash the towels, rugs, bed linens, or other items immediately by putting them in a washing machine. Be sure to use detergent, stain remover, and hot water. Wash your hands when you are finished. Use an antibacterial spray to mask remaining odors. These are difficult tasks; congratulate yourself for accomplishing them every time you do them.

Sharing Private Times

"It's like we can't get 'synced up' for sex," says David, 66. "One minute I might be interested, but she's just taken medication or is feeling nauseated. Then she might be feeling better and I'm so tired I can hardly make it to the bedroom. And of course I'm worried if I'm going to hurt her or seem selfish by even trying. But she tells me she wants to and needs to feel close to me, so we will keep trying."

Private times – treasured times that you spend with your partner, your special someone, your spouse – add color and dimension to everyday living. Feeling appreciated, wanted, and loved are important needs that should not be overlooked or avoided.

When you're caring for your partner, you'll probably have many questions about what's appropriate in terms of being intimate. Intimacy in the forms of touching, massage, and kissing is encouraged through all phases of treatment. Sexual intercourse, though, may be painful or difficult for a variety of reasons and communication may be strained. While your partner may not feel lovable because of a change in her appearance, you may not know how to touch her or talk to her about intimacy. The caregiver must be extra supportive and sensitive and the patient must be extra communicative and understanding. Encourage each other. You were partners before this illness made you patient and caregiver. You both need the strength from a loving relationship during treatment times.

Try to get together when you're both feeling pretty good. Rare as those moments are, they can happen between treatments (or cycles of treatments) when you've had some rest. Sexual positions may sometimes need to be changed or activity may need to be limited. Partners may need to find different tools or ways to pleasure each other. You may need to plan more than usual. No situation is perfect and there will sometimes be rejection. But taking the first step will provide something that you can build on later.

A Few Words on Pregnancy

Oncologists and fertility experts usually recommend that both patient and caregiver avoid trying to become pregnant during cancer treatment. Anti-cancer agents can cause damage to the chromosomes in sperm and children conceived during chemotherapy may suffer genetic damage. Ask a gynecologist and obstetrician for advice on the timing of chemotherapy or radiation if the patient is already pregnant when she is diagnosed.

Juggling Work Responsibilities

"Work? My job is getting the patient better," says Molly, 59. "There's no more important work than that. But, I have to admit, my other work is a welcome diversion sometimes."

Making the decision to continue working through treatment is difficult for both you and the patient. Most patients choose not to work during treatment but many caregivers do. Because your focus is caring for the patient, you may also be concerned about keeping your job. Cancer treatment can impact work productivity and attendance dramatically. Unfortunately, some employers regard absences or need for flexibility as a lack of commitment to work. Caregivers cite examples of being passed over for assignments or promotions because they can't be counted on to be there. As a result, caregivers and the patients find themselves faced with a difficult dilemma: how to provide an explanation for the change in their behavior and the need for flexibility without negative repercussions, including the loss of their jobs.

If either of you is working and wants to keep your job, you must be careful to schedule treatments within the limits of your work schedule and communicate that with appropriate personnel at work. The reaction of your co-workers will play a big part in your desire to share details by their reactions to them, so be selective. You need to make a plan about how to communicate.

The benefits administrator can provide you with some guidance on what flexibility and benefits may be offered by the government and supported by the company.

Changing Spiritual Perspectives

"The nerve," says Diane, 62, whose partner has been diagnosed with melanoma. "We used to be so close to God. Does he have something better to do than to listen to us?"

A person's relationship with a higher power is a private one. However, with the diagnosis of a serious illness, spirituality can take on a very public display in patients. Many will become stronger or more active in their current practice of faith. Others will experience a more drastic change. Formerly devout patients may suddenly turn their backs on religion, blaming a higher power for what is happening to them. Alternatively, the opposite may happen in patients who previously had little or no spiritual belief yet turn to a practice of religion for support and strength.

The more time you spend with the patient, the more likely you will see some of these changes. These are sometimes very painful to witness. As caregiver, you can continue to help him through changing spiritual perspectives by actively discussing his concerns. Try not to be judgmental if what he is doing or thinking spiritually is different from what you do or think. Bringing in trained social workers or spiritual/religious professionals is a good way to help you address unanswered questions or to resolve spiritual conflicts.

Taming the Impossible Patient

*"It doesn't seem fair," said Marie, 70. "I volunteered to take
care of him. No one told me that I was going to be on the
defensive all the time. I feel like I have to deflect his emotions
to protect myself. He lashes out as if I were the one causing
the cancer, not as though I'm trying to be part of the cure. At
this point, I'd much prefer the silent treatment."*

Not every patient is a model patient. Dealing with treatment outcomes
can't be easy on the patient. But it does not justify abusing the
caregiver.

Caregivers have to deal with emotional outbursts, hurtful comments,
accusations, and confessions just because they are nearby. If this is
your situation, you may need some ideas on what to do. To tame
the impossible patient, first nail down what it is that makes him
impossible to deal with. Is he:

- Ambivalent
- Angry, hostile
- Argumentative, moody
- Demented, doesn't recognize you
- In denial
- Entitled, demanding

- Diagnosed with other mental or personality disorders
- Manipulative, self-destructive
- Seductive or playful
- Silent or non-communicative
- Unappreciative
- Uncooperative or stubborn
- Violent.

Try not to react to his moods. You will probably have more success
if you take away known stressors. Keep mental notes on what
triggers outbursts and avoid them. Decide what can be managed by
empathizing and foster an alliance. Caregiving can be less taxing if
you use words like "I would probably feel the same way" or "Why
don't we try it another way?" Sometimes "I don't know what to say"
can be the perfect thing to say.

When you feel the need to argue or to speak bluntly to the patient, you probably need to carefully select the words that actually come out of your mouth. It's OK to be upset. Handling an impossible patient is very difficult, but consider the aftermath of saying something hurtful. Will you accomplish what you want, or will you just make things more tense? Only you can decide.

A Few Words on When to Stop

You may decide that enough is enough and it's time to quit being a primary caregiver. When the patient acts out against you, actively works against treatments or professionals, or doesn't complete his responsibilities, it is a recipe for failure. Caregiver effectiveness hinges on treatment consistency. Without the patient's cooperation during the course of treatment, caregivers feel angry, inferior, defeated, resentful, and abused. There are no standards on patient response; only you must determine what your breaking point is. Don't be afraid to walk away if it is emotionally or physically breaking you.

If you decide to continue giving care, there are concrete suggestions for a few more situations in the chart below.

Handling Challenging Patient Scenarios

Situation	How Can I Help?
Claims to be forgetful or has difficulty with mental clarity	• Mental clarity and memory may fluctuate with certain treatments. As healing occurs and fewer medications are introduced into the system, former mental abilities usually return. Have him write things down and keep his mind active with memory games or crosswords. Limit his decision-making.
Moods shift rapidly	• Determine the timing or cause of the patient's mood changes. If you find the stressors, avoid them. There are also medications for pain, anxiety, sleeplessness, or depression that may treat it.

Situation	How Can I Help?
Is angry and feels victimized. Normal struggles seem blown out of proportion.	• Encourage the patient to get more rest, as fatigue plays a role in this. You may need to be direct with him by giving some timely advice of: "You are not a victim." Help him feel empowered by reminding him of what he can do for himself. The more he can do for himself, the greater his sense of control.
Screams, yells, attacks, or insults you. Patient has low overall tolerance and so do you.	• Think of the insults as fastballs. They are pitched at you to be dodged or swung at, but don't get hit personally because they hurt. You may need to ignore some comments, strike back with a snappy retort, or respond with ground rules that you set for the patient. Start general conversation, asking about his day. Actively listen. If he starts arguing, see if there is any validity in what has been said. Take frequent breaks and keep a fresh outlook. Don't be afraid to set limits on your availability if most interactions are argumentative.
Drinks alcohol to excess or takes unauthorized medicines for comfort.	• Is the patient still wrestling with denial? Have a talk with him about the seriousness of the problem. Ask him if he knows he's doing this and involve a counselor or therapist if you are unable to reach him.
Rejects care or medicine.	• Hostile or aggressive behavior may reflect the feeling of helplessness and lack of control. Start by describing the care or the medicine by telling what it is and why it's needed. Consider alternatives that he suggests.
Patient gets violent.	• In violent situations, try not to be alone with the patient. Be aware of clothing or jewelry that can be used as a weapon. Put away anything that would inflict harm on either of you, such as guns, knives, or scissors. Involve a social worker or therapist if you're unable to manage this yourself.

Lassoing Stress with Complementary Therapies

When you're searching for relief from emotional distress, you and the patient may want to try these relaxation and stress prevention techniques. In some cases, you will need to find a teacher or a class. Many you can do on your own or with a book.

- Art Therapy – You may find solace in painting, drawing, sculpting, airplane modeling, quilting, or crafting. Local listings in newspapers, at schools, on television, or on the internet will help you to find classes or facilities.

- Exercises – Stretching and repetitive exercises, including sexual activity, will help tone, strengthen, and work tension away from the body. It will also promote healing and calmness. Look into a local health club or gym.

- Laugh Therapy – With laughter therapy, some swear that you are able to find energy when you're spent, find motivation when you're down, or find resolution when you don't understand. A good comedy show could also distract your thinking for a while.

- Pets – Pets can bring a world of change to the patient. They let the patient leave the role of victim to become a caregiver to something else.

- Qi Gong – An Asian healing approach, Qi Gong is a combination of visualization, concentrated breathing, and energy transfer of the qi (life force) to the necessary destinations within the body. While some practice individually, others practice in a group setting. There are tapes or CDs of Qi Gong master recordings or classes taught by local masters.

- Saunas and Baths – Formally known as hydrotherapy, the activity of using water and steam to relax has been around for centuries. Watch the temperature of the water or the steam room to avoid being burned. Remember to re-hydrate by drinking plenty of water afterwards. Your civic center or health club may have these amenities.

- T'ai Chi – This ancient Chinese method of slow, rhythmic movements is said to relax both mind and body, while helping to improve circulation, posture, and self-defense. Working with a T'ai Chi instructor will help you better understand the movements. There are studios for martial and Eastern arts and health clubs also offer these classes.

- Yoga – Yoga classes featuring poses, movement series, and meditation appeal to all age groups at all levels of fitness. These are often divided into beginner and advanced levels. The majority of these poses are non-stressors and some suggest that these exercises help with pain management as well. Yoga studios or health clubs have a range of class offerings.

Caregivers also recommend small changes in routine that may lead to larger changes in life. Some examples are carpooling to work, avoiding people that make you uncomfortable, and spending more time with supportive friends.

Taking Care of Yourself

"At first, I was afraid to let anyone else be there in the hospital." says Betty, 70. "What would they think if something happened when I wasn't there? After the first few times of letting our son take him in, though, I got a little more comfortable and now we alternate. What a relief!"

When the patient is having treatments and your responsibilities at home escalate, it's time to call in the reinforcements – your Care Team.

First, let's have a little review. In Chapter 3, we talked about forming your Care Team. You've lined up those whom you can count on for assistance including close friends, family members, neighbors, and other volunteers. You may also have been pleasantly surprised by the kindness of new acquaintances. All these wonderful people and the patient's healthcare providers form your Care Team. They watch out for you and the patient.

Now let's get back to the subject at hand: delegation. Earlier in this chapter, we mentioned delegating some of the caregiving tasks. During treatment, it's difficult, if not impossible, to take them all on yourself. Knowing that you can trust others to do them is a terrific blessing. Lean on the members of your Care Team.

To delegate, identify what needs to be done and consider which member of your Care Team would be the best one to do it. Ask for assistance. Be understanding if they can't do it this time and ask someone else. Or, ask that person to do something else.

Don't forget the organizations specific to your patient's illness, houses of worship, senior services, and other groups that have volunteers to help. When you need help, you need help, and when you ask people for assistance, they often give it. Making a couple of phone calls is a good way to take care of yourself as well as the patient – and it could save hours of your time and decrease your stress from too many items on the To Do list.

Wrapping Up

It's the end of the chapter but chances are it's not the end of your daily challenges during treatment. You won't know exactly what symptoms are coming or when they will be coming, but you can plan for the common ones. Keep referring back to this section as symptoms arise for ideas on how to manage them. Try to keep your chin up – most outcomes of treatment are short-term.

Here are a few other points you can take from this chapter:

- There is no reason you should be abused by an impossible patient. Determine what makes him impossible and counter it, or get assistance in caring for the patient.

- Consider trying some complementary therapies to lasso runaway stress like warm baths and art therapy.

- Daily functioning can be a challenge. When necessary, bring in others from your Care Team to fulfill those responsibilities. Don't forget about the support services from organizations. Call on them if you can use them.

The next chapter will tackle issues that surface after treatment has completed. Building on your new expertise in managing expected outcomes, we'll address other potential changes that may come at that time.

When treatment is finished, you'll both have reason to recover.

Chapter 8: Recovering and Managing After Treatment

"We're getting closer to the end of the tunnel," says Elaine, 56, whose husband is fighting prostate cancer. "I can see the light. I can see new life!"

Caregiver, you're terrific. We started this journey just a few chapters ago, learning about the roles of a caregiver and possible impacts to your lifestyle. You've taken on those roles and experienced the daily challenges that accompany the DIAGNOSIS and the treatment. Congratulations on having the endurance to continue on.

The goal of this chapter is to familiarize you with what may happen when all primary treatment prescribed for the patient has happened. That means all surgeries have happened and all prescribed doses of CHEMOTHERAPY and radiation have been given to the patient. With healthcare providers, this is called *post-treatment.*

When we say *post-treatment* in this book, we also mean the period of time after the procedure or treatment. That could be immediately or later – in some cases months or years after the treatment. If you have questions about the length of time that a post-treatment occurrence is happening, ask the patient's medical professionals.

In Chapter 8, we will talk about:

- Common Post-Treatment Occurrences

- Post-Treatment Check-ups

- The Need for Treatment Change

- Taking Care of Yourself.

You're in the home stretch. Let's continue by exploring what happens immediately after a treatment.

Understanding When Treatment Has Finished

"I think we're done with treatment for now," says Kelly, 39, who cares for his mother with lung cancer. "They say they caught it pretty early and it looks promising. I'm hoping they're right. I'd never tell her this, but I could use a break from all this too."

As a partner in the treatment process, you've likely been involved in the decision-making and the preparation surrounding it. And, if you've waited hours for radiation, spent time in the hospital after major surgery, or followed someone undergoing six months of chemo, you may even feel like you've experienced the treatment yourself. It's OK if you, like Kelly in the quote above, feel as if you could use a break.

You may also feel that you need some general advice after treatment ends. Each traditional treatment brings a specific set of post-treatment occurrences, and these are detailed over the next several pages. However, there are a few general post-treatment activities that may encourage healing for most treatment types, which you'll find in the next checklist.

Checklist: General Healing After Treatment

☐	Always work with the medical professionals to get an understanding of your situation, both short-term and long-term. Prepare a short list of possible scenarios including what you need to do if they happen. By writing these, you will also know when it's important to call for help.
☐	Get one name and phone number of who to call with medical questions.

☐	Monitor what the patient does/doesn't eat and drink and the medications he does/doesn't take in relation to the range in doctor's orders. Make an effort to keep what he does consistent with what he's supposed to do. Alert the patient's doctor of the differences.
☐	Pay attention to any swallowing or speaking difficulty and tell your medical professional. Additional evaluation and therapy may be needed if these situations continue with the patient.
☐	Understand the patient's needs and medical professional's recommendations regarding activity. Rest is often necessary after most treatments to let the body start healing itself. After surgery though, the patient may need to increase activity at a certain point in the healing cycle. This activity is intended to counter deterioration of the muscle function due to lack of use.
☐	Slowly take on movements that are painful or difficult for the patient.
☐	Observe breathing patterns and changes in consciousness. Problems in taking breaths or drifting in and out of consciousness could point to a number of possible issues, many of which are serious.
☐	Take temperatures and record readings as recommended by the medical professionals. Watch for elevation of temperature as a sign of infection.
☐	Identify some "healing milestones" with the medical professionals so the patient can strive for these goals.

During this critical post-treatment period, it's always better to make the mistake of calling the patient's medical professionals with questions more often than you may need to. It's easier to treat a serious problem if it's detected early. The sections that follow will help set your expectations about common occurrences after traditional treatments.

Anticipating Post-Treatment Occurrences

These next sections cover common post-treatment occurrences for surgery, radiation, chemotherapy, and a few other treatment types. They contain a lot of information, which may not sink completely in at one sitting. Read and re-read the sections as needed. You may want to skip some of these sections if they do not apply to the patient's situation. However, you may be interested in multiple sections if:

- Treatments prescribed by your medical professional are MULTIMODAL.

- The patient is fighting multiple sites of cancer, such as a primary TUMOR and METASTASIS.

- There is RECURRENCE of the cancer and additional treatment is required.

The important thing to remember about each treatment is its original purpose, so that you can gauge its success against that purpose. Let's take a look at each one.

Surgery

"We were calm and never pessimistic," says Mary Francis, 42, as her uncle approached surgery for gastric cancer. "We had confidence in our other doctors and our surgeon and I think this helped in recovery."

Going into the surgery, the procedure has probably been explained to you and you have probably discussed the risks and potential complications. You've also probably talked about any anticipated changes in body functions as well as survival results/statistics. So when it's time for surgery, you and the patient have an idea of what will take place and what to expect when it is finished.

Immediately after surgery, the surgeon will give you the following information (shown here with examples):

1. Patient's status (He's OK and he's in the ICU.)

2. What they found during surgery and what they did to respond to that (Tumor was larger than showed on scans, but we successfully took it out.)

3. What they found and did that was consistent with or deviated from the assessment or operating plan going in (It took us a little longer than planned. We had to work around a major vein, but it went just fine.)

4. Recovery expectations and when you can see the patient (Short-term, he will be in ICU for three days; long-term, he will be able to go home within a couple of weeks. He should be waking up within the hour. The final PATHOLOGY REPORT will be released by the end of the week and we'll make plans for follow-up care accordingly.)

5. An opportunity to ask any questions.

If you don't hear these things from the surgeon, gently ask for the information. Outcomes from surgery may vary because of many factors such as the type of surgery, the magnitude of the operation, the patient's underlying health, and the impact of any other major illnesses.

You may remember that with smaller operations patients usually recover faster than in larger/open surgeries. Open operations usually involve large incisions and require long recovery times. Even though the techniques of surgery may be different, the complications and healing processes may be similar.

In both types of surgery, tissue is removed and reviewed in the hospital's pathology lab. The pathologists, specialists in evaluating tissues and cells, examine the tissue and detail their findings. This Pathology Report describes the TUMOR-NODE-METASTASIS (TNM) features of the tissue according to the American Joint Commission on Cancer Guidelines®, including:

- Size and extent of the tumor

- Involvement of other adjacent organs

- Special features including involvement of NODES (with number and location)

- Presence of metastasis and significance of location (as related to SURVIVAL RATES)

- Complete or incomplete removal of the tumor (if MARGINS of the specimen showed tumor cells).

From the Pathology Report (and the findings at surgery or in imaging tests), the surgeon has evidence that supports any need for further treatment in the form of additional surgery, chemotherapy, or radiation. The surgeon should review the findings of the report with you and cover additional treatment needs and potential complications.

Complications

We have already covered the common effects that are treated in the care facility and those that could be managed at home with little or no difficulty. Other complications that may require increased medical attention and treatment are (listed in alphabetical order):

- Blood clots, particularly in the leg or in the pelvis, often after abdominal or pelvic surgery

- Increased problems of pre-existing illnesses or conditions

- Increased pain, redness, or drainage from the incision

- Pneumonia or ASPIRATION

- Prolonged nausea and vomiting

- Severe abdominal cramping and bloating

- Sudden swelling of arms and legs.

The hospital staff will take care of these symptoms while the patient is there. When the patient is ready to go home, the surgeon or staff member should talk to you about any remaining symptoms, so you will be able to manage them yourself. Don't be afraid to take notes or repeat back what you have heard. As you know, you'll be responsible for this care at home. If you see or suspect that the patient experiencing any of these major difficulties at home, call your key medical professional as soon as possible. They may ask you to bring the patient back to the emergency room, where he may possibly be re-admitted.

Radiation Therapy

"I'll have to admit, I was skeptical about her having radiation," says Marty, 68. "But it was amazing in terms of helping my sister's bone cancer pain. They said that was our best option and we went with it. I'm glad for her sake that we did."

RADIATION THERAPY has proven helpful in destroying CANCER CELLS, in shrinking tumors, and in decreasing cancer-related pain. However, it can cause damage to healthy cells in the radiated area and nearby structures such as tissues, organs and bones. The LATE EFFECTS of radiation can be particularly challenging: it has been shown to cause secondary cancers and secondary diseases that may surface years after treatment.

Therefore, like surgery, it's important to discuss the treatment with the medical professional (radiation oncologist, ONCOLOGY nurse or the nurse practitioner). The procedure has probably been explained to you, and you've probably discussed the risks and complications, anticipated changes in body functions, and survival results/statistics. So when it's time for radiation, you and the patient have an idea of what will take place and what to expect when it is finished. This applies to both single dose and multiple doses.

Immediately after radiation, the patient's radiation oncologist or attending nurse will give you the following information (shown here with examples):

1. Patient's status (She's OK and she'll be ready to go home soon.)

2. When you can see the patient (She should be waking up within the hour.)

3. Discharge instructions (You can expect her to have swelling and inflammation around the site, but if it becomes severe, contact us.)

4. Recommendations about close contact with the patient (She may need to avoid contact with others immediately after some forms of this treatment.)

5. An opportunity to ask any questions.

If you don't hear these things from the attending professional, gently ask for the information. Radiation is a serious treatment. You will want to be prepared for how to interact with the patient after therapy.

As mentioned before, the late effects of this procedure may sometimes appear years after treatment and a series of specialists may need to be involved in the patient's care as time goes on. Those who experience radiation to the throat, head, neck, and face may want to consider following up with visits to dentists to help heal and restore any damage to the mouth, gums, teeth, and jawbones. Those interested in having (more) children and who have experienced radiation to the abdomen may want to consider visiting fertility specialists, obstetricians/gynecologists and urologists to help them heal. These specialists can present options for conceiving, considering the late effects of the treatment.

Complications

We have already covered the common effects that are treated in the care facility and those that could be managed at home with little or no difficulty. Other complications that may require increased medical attention and treatment are (listed in alphabetical order, followed by the corresponding radiated area):

- Damage or dryness to walls of vagina (pelvis)

- Cataracts or tear gland dysfunction (eyes)

- Fibrous tissue (fibrosis) continuing over years (pelvis/uterus)

- Glandular dysfunction (throat/thyroid, upper and lower abdomen/ovaries and testes)

- Infertility (damage to tissues in and around sex organs)

- Osteoporosis or bone death, called osteoradionecrosis, when small blood vessels around the site are damaged and cannot bring blood to area (bones)

- Permanent hair loss (scalp)

- Permanent voice loss (head and neck)

- Premature menopause in women, including hormone changes, hot flashes, anxiety, sleep disruption (pelvis)

- Rotting teeth, receding gums, mouth sores, dry mouth (mouth, head, neck, and face)

- Temporal Mandibular Joint (TMJ) dysfunction (mouth, head, neck, face).

Most oncologists will recommend a series of check-ups after the radiation to monitor the patient for SIDE EFFECTS. Additional specialists may be consulted or other treatment options may be discussed at that time, according to the patient's situation.

Chemotherapy

"Who would have thought she would get 'chemo brain'?" *says Rodney, 48, whose wife is fighting indolent Non-Hodgkin's lymphoma. "She was always smarter than me! The doctor says enjoy to this while it lasts, because she'll be back in that position in no time."*

Chemotherapy may be prescribed a number of different ways, depending on the patient's needs. Therefore, like surgery and radiation, it's important to discuss the treatment with the medical professional (oncologist, oncology nurse or the nurse practitioner). The procedure has probably been explained to you, and you've probably discussed the risks and complications, anticipated changes in body functions, and survival results/statistics. So when it's time for the chemotherapy, you and the patient have an idea of what will take place and what to expect when it is finished. This applies to both single dose and multiple doses.

Soon after a particular session of chemotherapy, the oncologist or attending nurse will give you the following information (shown here with examples):

1. Patient's status (She's OK and she'll be ready to go home soon.)

2. What they did that was consistent with or deviated from the prescribed chemo REGIMEN going in (We used the standard regimen and we'll follow up with her prescription of prednisone.)

3. Recovery expectations (In the first dose, she'll be fatigued. We may make adjustments to the doses after we see how the cancer reacts to this first course. She probably won't lose any hair until the second or third week.)

4. When your next appointment/dose or blood count check will be (We need to set up a time next week for these.)

5. An opportunity to ask any questions.

If you don't hear these things from the attending professional, gently ask for the information. You will want to be prepared for how to interact with the patient after therapy.

Complications

We have already covered the common effects that are treated in the care facility and those that could be managed at home with little or no difficulty. Other complications that may require increased medical attention and treatment are (listed in alphabetical order, but divided by commonality):

More Common

- Premature menopause or menopausal symptoms, including hormone changes, hot flashes, anxiety, sleep disruption

- Reproductive damage, up to and including infertility or sterility.

Less Common

- Damage to the brain, liver, heart, or kidneys

- Secondary cancers including leukemias and myelodysplasias

- Serious difficulties in breathing including needing breathing assistance through a ventilator.

When any of these impacts happen, there may be the need to contact the patient's medical professionals for additional assistance. For example, the oncologist may be alerted by the lab analyzing the blood sample if there is possible significant impact on the BLOOD COUNTS and bone marrow of a cancer patient (especially in lymphomas and leukemias), requiring blood transfusions, antibiotics, or blood cell growth factors that will be scheduled with the chemotherapy. Total body (SYSTEMIC) support is available in different medications that help the body heal through rebuilding the white and red blood cells. Work with your oncologist to determine if these apply to the patient.

As with radiation, post-treatment recommendations often include referrals to other professionals who can help you with specific challenges. Fertility specialists, endocrinologists, obstetricians/ gynecologists and urologists have been consulted to help men and women interested in having (more) children after having experienced chemotherapy. Those professionals also can present options for conceiving considering the significant side effects of chemotherapy. The patient may also need to work with nutritionists and to understand and counter these effects.

Anticipating Outcomes with Other Treatments

Immunotherapy, Tumor Biology, Antibody Therapy, and Clinical Trials

These therapies will vary per patient and the outcomes will vary as well. The possible combinations are numerous. You will need to work with the patient's medical professionals to anticipate and address possible outcomes.

Hormone Therapy

There are a variety of side effects that may accompany hormone therapy, depending on factors such as the hormones affected, the patient's age and the dosage taken. For men, commonly reported side effects are decrease in sexual desire, enlarged breasts, hot flashes, impotence, and osteoporosis. For women, commonly reported side effects include fatigue, hot flashes, mood swings, nausea, osteoporosis, and weight gain. Every case is different. Work with the patient's medical professionals to monitor the patient closely. They will help you determine the severity and countermeasures, as appropriate.

215

What Do I Say? Questions for the Medical Professionals after Treatment

"I think I must have said 'I'm sorry, but would you please explain it again? We didn't quite understand.' about a dozen times," says Julia, 72, whose husband is fighting pancreatic cancer. "I'm sure the surgeon thought we were just dense, but he explained it until we got it."

Being prepared for phone calls or visits with medical professionals can help you to be an effective advocate for the patient and to get you the answers you need. Once again, you may need to brace yourself to ask some hard questions and to hear answers that are difficult, painful, or uncertain. Questions in this section may be a good start. Remember, there are no silly or stupid ones. These people are here to help you and they've probably heard your question before.

General Information

- When will the results be ready?

- What do the results mean? Did the treatment do what it was supposed to do?

- What about follow-up procedures, prescriptions, tests, check-ups?

- When can the patient go back to work, being intimate, exercising?

- Do we have any special nutritional concerns?

- If we have questions later, who should we call?

- To whom should I direct insurance claim questions?

Presence of Cancer

- We are afraid. What could we do to try to overcome this?

- If the cancer is gone, how likely is it to come back?

- What are the signs to watch for recurrence? When should we call your office?

- What changes are *not* signs of recurrence? When should we *not* call your office?

- If the cancer is not gone, where is it? What's next?

- We know that there are common links between some cancers. How (and when) do we test for other cancers, if at all?

<u>Fertility Options</u>
- When can we start trying to have a family again?

- How likely is it that we can conceive, have a healthy pregnancy, and have a healthy baby at this point?

- Who are the specialists that we can talk to about trying to conceive and what should we do if we encounter problems?

- How do we follow up with you?

Your follow-ups will be guided by the medical professionals. These are generally called Post-Treatment Check-ups. We'll explain them and help you prepare for them within the next few sections.

Handling Post-Treatment Check-Ups

"We wanted to go back to the doctor. We wanted to show him how well we healed, both of us," said Mike and Tammy, each 60, who were fighting early stage prostate cancer in Mike. "We were stronger than the cancer and we wanted everyone to know it."

Although they are not part of the daily routine, check-ups are important parts of treatment. Each type of treatment requires some follow-up care, even if it's simply an affirmation that the patient is healing well.

The post-treatment check-ups usually occur some weeks after the procedure and take place in the specialist's office. The patient is examined, questions are asked, and more comparison tests or scans may be ordered to establish a new baseline (status of the patient's progress today) and to look for recurrence. Most patients (and many caregivers) don't want to go to check-ups. The hospital or office sounds and smells can be upsetting and nauseating, bringing back painful memories. It may be hours until you see the medical professional. The patient may feel branded as a cancer patient and you may feel branded as the family or the friend of the cancer patient. No matter how good the patient is looking or feeling, you carry these titles in the healthcare world. And, to top it all off, there is always the chance of bad news. More treatment. More tests. More x-rays or scans. More painful procedures. *More cancer.*

But check-ups are necessary. What you can get out of the check-ups are:

- Peace of mind that the treatment was successful

- Understanding of what is normal, and consistent with what's happening for the patient's age, type of cancer, type of treatment, and current state of health

- Plan for continuing care (including direction on ending or refilling prescriptions).

Check-Up Expectations

It's helpful if you know what else to expect from the check-ups. The medical professionals (primarily the physician) will perform a physical examination, discuss any ongoing symptoms, review any recent test results and doctor's notes, and plan the next steps of care. The physician will let you know when you need to schedule your next check-up, as well as the need for ongoing tests, such as:

- Scans (CT, MRI, bone scan, chest x-rays, mammograms)

- Gastro-intestinal studies, including colonoscopies

- Physical exams and blood tests

- Routine health maintenance. For women, this means gynecologic exams, pap smears, monitoring of menopausal symptoms, and vaginal sonograms. For men, this means digital rectal exam and Prostate Specific Antigen (PSA) level for the prostate.

You should encourage but not force the patient to schedule and go to the appointments. If it is clear that the patient needs a little nudging to go, try to offer the support to make that happen. If it is clear that the patient will not go, call the office and cancel the appointment.

After you've decided to go to the check-ups, you and the patient can do several things to prepare.

Step 1: Schedule the appointments at the correct intervals.

Step 2: Decide who will drive. Have a backup person lined up if you need a break. You can delegate driving to these appointments to others who want to help.

Step 3: Make sure to bring the patient's MEDICAL HISTORY with you. With surgery, the surgeon may request that the patient keeps a symptom notebook, food diary, or a log of drainage for a tube. If so, chart the items and bring the documents to discuss.

Step 4: Share the treatment information with all the patient's medical professionals. Have the necessary reports and papers ready. These professionals need to know what's going on and they may not know if the patient has had treatment elsewhere.

Step 5: Keep the medical professionals informed of good things that happen (like her hair is growing back) as well as other symptoms that concern you.

Step 6: Relax. It will make the check-ups go more smoothly.

Checklist: Evaluate a Post-Treatment Check-Up

After the patient's check-up, you may find yourself evaluating if it was good or not. You may want to tell others how it went, so you'll need to form your response to them.

Try not to evaluate check-ups as successful if there is little or no evidence of cancer and unsuccessful or bad if there is more cancer or if more treatment is needed. Try instead to evaluate check-ups the way outlined in the checklist that follows.

☐	I understood the status of what's happening with the patient.
☐	We've got the information we need.
☐	We've planned the next steps together.
☐	I'm comfortable with what to expect in the immediate future.
☐	Our immediate quality of life is a concern for the medical professionals.
☐	I know who to call if I have questions or need to schedule another appointment.

If you can check all these boxes, the check-up was successful and you know what's likely to happen next. Good job. If you aren't able to check all those boxes, call the nurse and ask for what you need.

What Do I Say? Talking to Others about the Patient's Progress

There are many benefits involved in sharing your experience. Usually, as patients and caregivers prepare for treatment and live through the effects of treatment, there is much to discuss: treatment response, follow-up care, and changes in routine. Depending on your personality, you may tend to talk more than others (or not talk at all). Likewise, some people may want to hear about the patient's progress more than others (or not at all).

It may be difficult to interpret your listener's intentions and their responses. You may be able to identify their fears and insecurities because they may mimic your own. You may have a pre-set idea of how they will respond and they may not meet your expectations (such as not being as sympathetic as you would expect). Even after good news, you may hear their questions or comments as reminders of the fragility of health. As you are beginning to forget about the disease and its impacts to you, the rest of the world may not have caught up with you.

You may not always use the correct word to describe a precise situation and your listeners may not always respond correctly to the situation as described. This can be disappointing and hard to react to, but drum up some extra patience because they really do mean well and really do care (for the most part).

Some of the typical questions are included here. Think about how you want to answer common questions and remember: (1) Not all people want details of the trials and tribulations (or celebrations) and (2) It's always okay to say: "I just don't know right now, but I'll get back to you."

- **"How are things going? What's happening with the patient and how's she doing?"** – Many caregivers have found that there are times when they are just tired of talking about it. If you feel this way, politely say "Thanks for asking, but can we talk about something else for a while?" However, if you're comfortable talking about it, consider the listener's time and interest (as well as your time and interest) and respond accordingly. You can even suggest that they may want to call directly, if she is accepting outside calls.

- **"You've tried just about everything, haven't you? Can't they come up with anything that works?"** – No one needs to hear this defeatist attitude or patronizing comments like "You poor kid" or "Bless your heart." You may wonder how this helps you or anyone else. Try not to tell them where they can 'shove it.' Sometimes nodding your head and not responding is the best answer to those types of comments. Perhaps you can ask if they have any other suggestions or just ask them to keep you in mind and in their prayers.

- **"Sounds like you have some things to be happy about and celebrate."** – Everyone should have a moment or two to be joyous about. And if you're fortunate to have the patient be declared 'Free of Disease' or 'No Evidence of Disease,' don't be afraid to shout it from the mountains: "We do have something to celebrate! We've won! We have our lives back! We are so incredibly thankful and blessed! We feel like singing!" You deserve it.

- **"Good, you get a chance to rest now."** – Without one or several caring responsibilities claiming your time, you might have a chance to catch up on sleep and if you do, take advantage of it. To answer them, though, perhaps you should use something vague such as "I guess we could all use a good night's sleep" and let it be at that.

- **"Aren't you afraid it will come back? What's the likelihood of recurrence?"** – This is another highly emotionally-charged area. The nerve of the people asking – how could they, when you're attempting to enjoy one good thing that happened? Try not to see this as a validation of your own questions and fears. However, you should readily discuss these matters with the medical professionals and be armed with responses for when you choose to share the information. While recurrence is always a possibility, it doesn't always have to be a topic of conversation. Most likely, those asking will have a strong interest in you or the patient. When you're ready, talk about it honestly with the medical professionals, so that they can help you prepare if this happens.

A Few Words on Patients Not Wanting the Attention to End

There are occurrences when the patient does not want the care and attention to end. Some patients may exaggerate or fake their symptoms (especially pain or nausea, which are not seen outwardly). They may do so because they enjoy the attention or they don't want to return to their own responsibilities. You need to find out which complaints are real and which are exaggerated. Don't be afraid to get a second opinion and follow up accordingly.

Facing a Change in Treatment Plan

When a course of treatment is prescribed, the goal is always to get through treatments as quickly and as safely as possible. No one wants to endure more than necessary. Sometimes, though, if the patient is fighting multiple kinds of cancers or a recurrence of the same cancer, his original treatment plan may change.

It is often necessary to take extra steps to eliminate every trace of the cancer. These can come in the form of "more of the same" kind of treatment, such as another cycle of chemotherapy, a second surgery, additional radiation. Or the extra steps may come as a different treatment, such as surgery after radiation or radiation after surgery.

223

The standard practice is to create the entire plan before any treatment begins. That is, the first treatment is completed with the second treatment in mind. However, if the need for the second treatment is not recognized or not necessary when planning the first treatment, it may come as a shock or as a disappointment for both you and the patient.

After surgery, the surgeon/surgical oncologist will determine whether further treatment will offer any benefit in terms of controlling the cancer or decreasing the likelihood of its return. He may recommend ADJUVANT THERAPY, or additional treatment, after the removal of the tumor. This adjuvant therapy (usually radiation or chemotherapy) is administered to kill remaining cancerous cells that are not visible during surgery or by imaging tests (scans or X-rays).

As with surgery, the medical professional will determine whether further treatment will offer any benefit after radiation or chemotherapy. After radiation, surgery may be needed. After chemotherapy, radiation may be needed.

With any cancer, there is a possibility of developing a recurrence or METASTATIC disease. When there is further evidence of cancer, an evaluation is necessary to determine whether this is a recurrence of the original cancer or it is a new primary cancer. Then treatment is recommended accordingly.

It's easy to feel out of control with a second diagnosis or second recommendations on treating the cancer, especially when you are still reeling from an earlier treatment. Most patients will go through a prescribed treatment if they trust in the healthcare providers and know the repercussions if they do not, even if they do not understand the treatment itself. You may feel more in control if you understand what the options are and what the need for the next treatment is. Then you can make the decision together if you want to proceed or not.

In certain cases, you may think that the additional treatment is not worth it; that the risk outweighs the benefits. Don't be afraid to ask questions of another oncologist (for a second opinion), or tap into other organizations specific to your cancer concern for more information.

The hope for all patients is successful primary treatments resulting in strong survivorship. Sometimes, that is not the case. It can be necessary to follow multiple treatments before strong survivorship. In some cases, patients will try the three traditional curing methods but still have no success in curing the disease. If you and the patient are faced with progressive cancer after surgery, radiation and chemotherapy, take heart: we devote an entire handbook to care options that you do have. To find *The Compassionate Caregiver's Handbook on Hospice and Palliative Care,* go to www.compassion atecaregiveronline.com.

Taking Care of Yourself

> *"I've been experiencing a lot of indigestion and abdominal pain lately. I think it's just because of the stress," says Tripp, 40, whose wife has been diagnosed with gastric cancer. "Or, it could be sympathy pains. If it doesn't stop, I'll get it checked when she's all better."*

While Tripp thinks he's doing a service to his wife, he may not be especially if he's facing a serious health concern of his own.

Instead, Tripp should consider doing a short health assessment. As his wife is going to treatments and post-treatment check-ups, he should reflect on his own need for medical care. He should take the time for a short exam by his family doctor to do an overall health check-up. There he could discuss any symptoms he's been having and understand the severity of the symptoms. They could be nothing to worry about or they could be worrisome, and after talking to the medical professional he will know how to address them.

It's important to regularly do your own health check. Don't think of it as another item on your To Do list that you don't have time for. Think of it as part of giving good care. If you must, call it a responsibility to the patient. If something happens to you, where will that leave her? Take a minute and check yourself out. You're allowed to do this.

Ask your primary care doctor for a referral to an internist or family practice physician in the same medical community (facility or campus) where the patient will be treated. After you find a physician there, schedule an appointment near the time that the patient is having treatment, so you can have your exam when she's already planning to be there. Instead of waiting in the office, you can get a short exam done and usually be back before the patient needs to go home.

A health check-up is pretty simple. Usually during a physical exam, the doctor or nurse will check your blood pressure, listen to your heart and your breathing, and check your weight. They will listen to you explain any unusual symptoms or concerns, so before you go, take an inventory of your current condition. How are your eyes, skin, hair, muscles, bones, and heart, doing? Does anything need some attention? If you become aware of something that seems more serious or highly irregular, make a note of it. Then take a look at the mental and emotional. Does anything need some attention there? If so, ask for a referral to a therapist or professional when you're getting your exam. It's better to be safe than sorry, as the saying goes. Getting a physical exam could put your mind – and any ailments – at ease.

Wrapping Up

Think back to when we began this chapter. It may seem years ago! You were probably a little nervous about what would happen after the patient's primary treatment has stopped.

Having this information at your fingertips will give you a 24-hour reference. You should have a better idea about which common outcomes can be managed at home. You should also understand which require additional medical assistance. You're not alone and don't be afraid to reach out. Call the nurse or other medical professional if you're having difficulty with managing symptoms. We are getting through this!

A few other points that you may pull from this chapter are:

- There are many ways to promote a patient's healing, no matter which treatment she has.

- You can evaluate a post-treatment check-up other ways than just the news itself. Think about the patient's overall health and quality of life.

- It's important for you to recover as well. You need to schedule a regular check-up for yourself and discuss personal symptoms or concerns with the medical professional.

Next we'll look at living as survivors. With the ability to manage more daily challenges that may surface after treatment, you'll be able to make new habits that are part of healthy survivorship.

Chapter 9: Living as Survivors

"We decided we're going for long-term survivorship," says Bernie, 84, with a chuckle. "We've beat her cancer this far!"

Congratulations! You're approaching the end of your caregiving journey. More and more people are living successful, healthy lives after cancer treatment. They are survivors. To promote the possibility of long-term survivorship in your situation, we're going to start calling the cancer patient the *cancer survivor.*

The goal of this chapter is to equip you with solutions to problems that sometimes surface in the survivor after treatment and get you ready for a new routine as your responsibilities change. We will use this chapter to discuss:

- Becoming a Survivor

- Mastering Challenges in Daily Living – Part II

- Celebrating With the Survivor

- Creating a New Role for You

- Defining Goals for Healthy Living

- Taking Care of Yourself.

Some post-treatment issues can be highly complex and sensitive, but we'll take a look at some of the common ones in a simplified way. These may be tough, but we're with you until the end. The next section will help you understand what it means for the patient to become a survivor.

Becoming a Survivor

> *"Some people called him a 'survivor' on the day of his diagnosis, which didn't make sense to me but it was a good motivator for us," says Pedro, 55. "Now he's done with treatment and been called Free of Disease. That's what I call survivorship!"*

When the patient was first diagnosed, survivorship may have seemed a long way away. On this journey, the patient has faced his own mortality, learned about the disease, become dependent on medical and non-medical caregivers, and had many tests and treatments. You have been with him many steps on the way. With the treatments coming to a close and the healing continuing it's time for the patient to make the change.

Helping the patient move from being the victim (and the one who was waited on) to being the survivor (and the one who needs to re-embrace some level of independence) is a major transition. It's like rowing a boat – you have some of the activity but they do too. You need to agree on the goal and move together, in the same direction, for any kind of progress. The transition of becoming a survivor will be smoother when he understands his new roles and responsibilities.

What It Means to be a Survivor

Just as caregiving is not a responsibility to be taken lightly, cancer survivorship is not a responsibility to be taken lightly. For a short time after treatments, the survivor's sole responsibility should be healing. However, he will need to return to a life where he is doing as much as possible to help on that way to recovery and his own independence.

As a survivor, he has responsibility to watch over his own nutrition, to form healthy habits, and to follow the medical instructions to keep the disease in check. There will be short-term changes and long-term changes, many of them positive. It's up to the survivor to function with these, even though it may be difficult, and it's up to the survivor to ask for help if the situation requires it.

Unfortunately, as he transitions into that role, you may need to remind him of these things. The two sections that follow give you some suggestions on communicating with the survivor. Every day is a different day and moving into survivorship is challenging. A little awkwardness is to be expected, but stay flexible.

Talking to the Survivor

"You know, sometimes I just don't know what to say to him," says Malika, 40. *"It's like he is a different person after that surgery."*

Typically, healthcare providers give little training on survivorship. They give even less training to caregivers for communicating with the survivor. It's hard to know what to say and when. As we've said before, silence has its place, but after cancer treatment it's important to get a handle on how the survivor is feeling and what direction he sees his future taking.

You might start by talking about their priorities and what survivorship means to them. It's hard to bring these subjects up, but it's necessary. Then bring up how they see their lives changing. Ask what activities they will start doing or discontinue doing. You may get a couple of different answers. At first, you may hear an immediate, even glib, response but with introspection and more discussion, you may hear more involved responses. Before you act on anything he says, discuss it frequently to be sure that's what he really wants.

When you've been able to have some good discussions, give yourself credit for doing so. It's great that you're talking. That's taking a big step towards healing.

What Do I Say? Answering Questions from the Survivor

After treatment, the survivor may ask some hard questions that you will not be trained to answer. It's OK to say you don't know and to search out some solutions: explore the internet, participate in support groups, or ask the medical staff for recommendations.

You can't be expected to know everything. Concentrate your efforts on what you can help with. Here are some phrases to answer common questions and promote good conversation. You may need to alter the responses based on your situation, but just reading them may decrease the possibility of having to "answer on the fly."

- **Why am I still here? What does the future hold?** – It's difficult to find anyone who knows the answer to these questions. But this is a chance to talk through what has meaning in life and how this second chance can be used to make a difference in other's lives.

- **When can I go back to work/make love/give a piggy-back ride to my kids/golf?** – An ongoing discussion with the medical professionals will help you determine when it's safe to begin normal activities. After treatment, they may have to make some modifications such as working from home, trying different approaches to intimacy, skipping with your kids instead of carrying them, using a cart instead of walking the golf course. Keep trying and be creative!

- **Since I've had cancer, how will I date/be sexually active/find someone to marry/have children?** – These are tender topics. Sometimes the best approach is to listen. The current approach in medicine is to rely on a team of people to work through questions and problems. This team may include urologists (for men), obstetricians/gynecologists (for women), social workers, and relationship therapists. Chaplains or other spiritual leaders may also be suggested. There are social groups for cancer survivors, many of which may be found online. Take advantage of the resources that are available and don't be afraid to ask questions.

- **How do I answer 'How are you'?** – Be brief but truthful.

- **Will I have recurrence or will it develop somewhere else? I know now that my life and good health could all be taken away so quickly.** – There will always be fear of recurrence and METASTASIS. After a person has cancer, he is faced with his mortality and the possibility of death becomes real. Regardless of the treatment success or PROGNOSIS, the survivor will maintain that possibility of death. This is a subject that will probably surface a number of times; few tire of talking about it. Get information from the medical professionals. Tell him to try to focus on the survivorship statistics and on his new possibilities.

- **If I miss a day of exercise or don't watch my nutrition, will I be dead next year?** – This falls along the lines of knowing the future. Let the survivor know that you will talk about anything with him, but that neither of you know what definitively will be. It's up to him to try to maintain a healthy way of life.

Now that we have some communication situations handled, let's talk about challenges in your home and lifestyle.

Mastering Daily Challenges – Part II

It's almost impossible to categorize the many changes that may take place in the home after a survivor has completed treatment for cancer. As in Chapter 7, we've presented solutions to scenarios that nearly every caregiver will encounter in daily living:

- Managing Meals and Changing Nutritional Needs

- Moving, Washing, and Dressing the Survivor

- Sharing Private Times

- Juggling Work Responsibilities

- Changing Spiritual Perspectives.

Because you have likely come across these challenges during the patient's treatment, you may have an idea on how to approach them now. That's great. However, some curve balls can come at you after treatment. We'll go through these scenarios again so you can hit those curve balls right out of the ballpark.

Managing Meals and Changing Nutritional Needs

> *"I didn't understand why he was spending so much time in the bathroom after having chemotherapy," says Natalie, 45, whose husband was fighting osteosarcoma. "Then we found out he had sensitivities to different foods in addition to nausea and vomiting. It was hard for him to even try to eat."*

Cancer treatments often affect eating habits and there may be a period of adjustment for both you and the survivor. There will be some trial-and-error efforts about what does and does not work for the survivor. Don't be too hard on yourself. As the survivor heals, dietary needs will likely change and they may even return to pre-treatment times. In the meantime, here are some suggestions to counter common obstacles.

Handling Challenges With Meals and Nutrition

Situation	How Can I Help?
Survivor has new dietary restrictions.	Ask the medical professional (especially nutritionists and dieticians) to help with food recommendations. Wellness centers and support groups often share recipes and give cooking classes. Check the internet for suggestions, too.
Survivor (or you) cannot afford the special diet recommendations.	Investigate the financial support that is available through various agencies. Continue trying – it's important for the survivor to give his body the fuel it needs to heal.
Survivor has received recommendations for weight management (loss or gain).	It is difficult to help change the survivor's habits unless they want them to change. Be sure that he knows the impacts of the needed change and what the risks will be if the change doesn't happen. Work with him to find a starting point that will comply with his wishes and the doctor's guidance.
Survivor will not make needed changes to diet because of personal life.	Survivors may need some persuading that their diet really does impact the healing process. However, it may not be possible to change their diets or their minds. Understand your constraints and don't hurt yourself trying to change them.

With new day-to-day requirements for the survivor, you may find yourself taking a crash-course in food preparation or nutrition. Have faith: Even if cooking is not your favorite subject, you will learn what you need to know.

Moving, Washing, and Dressing the Survivor

"Her skin was so sensitive from the rashes after radiation,"
says Manuela, 78, whose daughter was fighting breast
cancer. "On top of that was the place where the surgery was.
She's sure it will leave a scar. It's so hard for her to raise her
arms or put on clothing, things we take for granted."

Outward signs of cancer treatment come in a variety of forms, from
sensitive skin to a change in bodily function. As previously discussed,
moving, washing, and dressing can present major challenges during
treatment. They can continue to present problems after treatment, as
the body heals and adjusts. You may witness that the survivor can't do
things the way she used to. She may need to modify how she walks,
how she cleans herself, and the clothing she wears. She may have
many needs that she did not have before the treatment.

Of the traditional treatments, surgery most often leaves behind an
outward reminder. If mechanical aids or prosthetics are necessary
– and many times they are – it can be difficult to adjust to them.
Breast forms, wigs, braces, or other appliances can be intimidating
and take some getting used to physically. Don't let the survivor take
on the changes alone. Use your wonderful communication skills to
connect her with relevant specialists or therapists. Let them guide
you with suggestions and shortcuts.

Also consider how the survivor is affected emotionally. If the
survivor's appearance is altered, part of the survivor's identity is
gone. In addition, people's reactions may be a reminder that surviors
are different or that they are sick. She will be off-key for a while,
having experienced a major trauma to her body. As a result, she may
feel self-conscious, unattractive and even anti-social. These feelings
can be hard to overcome. Train yourself and the survivor on ways
to increase her activity and her independence. Usually, the more
independent the survivor feels, the better her attitude. When that
happens, everyone's life runs a little more smoothly.

Sharing Private Times

"We asked our doctor about when we could resume our sexual relations after my husband's surgery. Instead of answering our question easily, he mumbled something. He was embarrassed and what he said was technical, not at all sensitive or helpful. He dismissed the subject and we left there thinking we shouldn't have even brought it up."

Most psychologists agree that major events cause people to evaluate different aspects of their lives and relationships are no exceptions. A major illness brings emotional impacts and physical changes that can test any relationship. When it brings resentfulness, frustration, and bitterness, it's sometimes hard to resurrect feelings of affection.

Regaining equilibrium in your relationship is a natural part of healing after treatment. Both caregivers and survivors may go through a grieving stage, which must be worked through before they begin to analyze their needs. It's important not to force the healing process. It's also natural to consider a change for the better. Let's take a look at the challenges with intimacy, sexuality, and fertility.

Intimacy Challenges

We will differentiate intimacy from sexuality by emphasizing that intimacy addresses the need for affection between two people, and it is not necessarily sexual. It can include touching, brushing the hair, kissing the face, massaging the shoulders, and washing or putting lotion on the body.

It's important for caregivers and survivors to remember the things they had in common. Amidst all the changes, most want to share thoughts and feelings. Most want some sense of closeness instead of growing apart. Most want some warmth and affection instead of rejection. Concerns from both of you become questions about the relationship, like:

> ➢ "I've emotionally grown apart from him. We have nothing to talk about now."

> "I share kinship with others who are experiencing same trauma. Other people I've met know what I've been going through."

> "He tells me that I'm not attractive to him any more. What do I do?"

> "Should we continue the same relationship/marriage or not? Is it worth it to continue dealing with the same problems for this current relationship and the additional ones brought on by the cancer?"

> "Is now the time to make a change? I've needed an excuse and now I've got one."

Divorce and separation/breakup are common after cancer DIAGNOSIS. They are even more common after treatment (some sources report up to 40%). Physical, spiritual, emotional, and financial stress can cause many people to stop the course of a relationship and to start something new and different. This is the right solution for some.

However, as the stress wanes and the treatments finish, there are additional changes. Many caregivers and their survivors report that there is a desire to forgive, to try again, and to remember the good in the relationship. The desire to be close often returns after treatments stop and healing is present. Feelings fluctuate over time – sometimes drastically. Trying again with the same relationship is the right solution for others.

As with any trauma, it is important not to act impulsively in your relationships or otherwise. There are opportunities to think about your situation and to decide what's right for you. Sometimes learning to talk about what you need is difficult and it may help to involve a third party if you can't seem to bring it up.

To address your own intimacy needs, you may want to work with a therapist, social worker, or spiritual leader. Wanting intimacy is natural and normal and you deserve it.

Sexuality Challenges

If the survivor is your parent, friend, or sibling, you may not have a sexual relationship. You may still want to read this to understand some concerns the survivor and his partner may have.

Believe it or not, both caregivers and survivors manage to think about intimacy and sexual activity while battling fatigue, trauma, and treatment recovery. They also voice concerns about sexual activity, including: too much change to deal with, too little activity, no interest, emotional and physical pain. These are common problems.

How you think about yourself as a sexual being is a primary element of sexuality. How you think about your partner as a sexual being is another and how you want to share those things with each other is the third. These three elements are basic but very complex. When you've both experienced the horrors that a cancer diagnosis can bring, it can be difficult to think of anything as sexual and desirable. You may be worried that there always is something else that needs to be done. One woman's words, "I know it's important, but can I get to it after I get some sleep?" sums up how many caregivers feel. Both of you may need the extra intimacy and release that accompany intercourse or other sexual activity.

Before your experience with cancer, there was normal pattern in your life. It came about because of factors in your life at that time: with whom, how much, when, and level of intensity. You and your partner may (or may not) want to return to that normal. You may want to alter it in some way because of the different set of factors in your life at this time, post-cancer treatment.

How can you start getting to a normal sexual pattern? Whether you want to return to your prior normal or a new one, each couple is different.

You might try these suggestions:

- Encourage each other. Give each other reasons to try new things together. Try to rediscover each other.

- Try to understand that neither partner wants this experience to be uncomfortable. It may take a little time to find out what works for both of you, especially if there are new physical considerations. While it's sometimes easier to concentrate on what used to be, try to appreciate what you do have and be creative.

- People may laugh, but sometimes writing down what you're thinking about will help to communicate what you need.

If you've been comfortable enough with the doctor, nurse or other medical professional to talk about these issues, you probably can continue the discussion. If not, there's no time like the present to start trying. These issues will not go away without communication. Try not to let your embarrassment or reluctance stop you from getting the answers you need. Know that the medical professionals have probably heard these questions before.

You're not alone in dealing with this. Other caregivers have been through sexual dilemmas after treatment too, and they describe their situations below. Although they may not match your situation, they may at least get you talking about what's going on with the two of you.

Handling Challenges With Sexuality

Situation	The partner is affected by the physical changes and is not interested in intercourse or intimacy.

"Does he honestly think I can think about sex when he has a colostomy bag connected to his insides? Besides being a physical bag between us – it's cold, looks awful and is sometimes slimy – it stinks and it makes me gag. I'm afraid no matter how careful we are it would rip right open. Then were would we be, with waste all over the place? Humiliating. And not even my idea! I would rather just stay away from it. Not even try."

How Can I Help?	Couples may try a variety of exercises to help get things started. Can you remember a time when you were attracted to him? How about reminiscing about a favorite sexual experience you shared? Is there a way to replay or re-enact what happened, even in a modified way? How can you relax and get comfortable together?
	Sometimes the effects of treatments heal and the survivor's former looks return. Feelings may also be altered over time. However, some changes are permanent and you need to make the decision if you can live a meaningful life together as it is or if you need to make a change. Talk to a therapist or other professional to help you work through your feelings and to make those choices. You owe it to yourself and to your partner to take time when making any major decision.

Situation	The survivor no longer feels desirable, feels unattractive or unwanted.

"My mother remarried after my father died. With her breast cancer, she had had a radical mastectomy and had a huge scar down the front of her. That was 30 years ago. It's much different today, but then it was dreadful. Even though I didn't like the guy she married, I knew that was what she needed to be whole again, to feel attractive and desirable after such a terrible ordeal."

How Can I Help?	Try to encourage physical contact and reconnection. If possible, take a vacation when both of you are physically and emotionally ready. Go to a health spa, gym, or any other place that is relaxing and away from any medical settings. In a loving way, ask what the specific concern is. For example, what she doesn't like about her body. Sometimes, you can help overcome her insecurities just by saying it's a part of her and you love every bit of her. You can also compliment something you've always loved that is unchanged or even enhanced. It may take some time or repetition, but keep trying.

Situation	The treatments have left a direct impact on the survivor so that mobility is temporarily or permanently changed.

"My boyfriend told me he was just as interested in getting back to our active sex life as I was but he needed a little time to heal. The colon surgery was pretty extensive and I think a 'little' is going to be a 'long' time. I mean, when you cut abdominal muscles, they need more than 'a little' time to heal. But the doctor said we could try a couple of different ways as soon as my boyfriend felt up to it. At least we can look forward to some variety."

How Can I Help?	When the survivor and the partner want to be held, feel close and cuddle, this should be possible in most situations. However, it may sometimes be medically inadvisable to attempt intercourse until the survivor has had some healing time. Ask your doctor when he's ready to go home.

Situation	The survivor has premature menopause.
"My fiancée changed into a demon. Crying, throwing things. It wasn't until I made a joke about 'hot flashes' that we finally realized there was a problem. The literature had mentioned menopausal symptoms and probably even the doctor said something, but we blew it off because we're only in our thirties. I thought you had to be in your fifties to experience that, but after she had radiation, it brought it on. And it wasn't pretty."	
How Can I Help?	Most of these symptoms can be controlled with medication and therapy. Ask your doctor about ways to counter this activity.
Situation	The male survivor is unable to have or maintain an erection or to ejaculate.
"I know there are ways we can be intimate, even though my husband is impotent from his prostate surgery. He doesn't even want to try. I even wonder if it's wrong that I still want sexual contact. Is it awful if I think about it?"	
How Can I Help?	Some medications cause temporary impotence, so talk to the doctor about this first. It could be just a matter of time before the drug works itself out of the system. If the situation seems linked with low testosterone levels, ask about him taking testosterone. Some other non-technology approaches have proved successful as well. Ask about performance-enhancing prescriptions or herbal approaches that have good research results. When impotence appears to be a permanent issue, consult an urologist to identify the best approach. If the survivor is willing to consider using technology, there are reputable products, such as pumps, semi-rigid implants and inflatable implants for lasting erections.

If you find that you just can't talk about sexuality concerns with anyone medical and you need more answers than what you've seen here, you might try reading a little. Many helpful books and articles are out there. You may also want to look at web sites to guide you. Sexual activity is a basic need for everyone and though it may take a little effort to get back on the saddle, it will probably be worth it for both of you.

Fertility Challenges

You and the survivor may not have the concerns about fertility if one or both of you are beyond child-bearing years. However, a cancer diagnosis in a survivor within child-bearing years often raises the question: "What about having (more) children?" With that, the pressure to make the decision about having or raising children is escalated. This is because one partner may be infertile, sterile, or unable to help raise the child as a result of cancer experience or treatments. Time may also be a concern, if the decisions about treatments need to be made immediately.

Discussions of conceiving and raising children can be complex even in the best of circumstances. When there is a serious illness to contend with, it tends to increase the emotional involvement for both people, especially if the caregiver and survivor are a couple. Additionally, the illness and its treatments can bring physical changes that become significant considerations if a couple is trying to conceive. In either gender, fertility may be impacted:

- If any part of the reproductive system is removed in surgery

- If the pelvic area or brain are radiated. In the pelvis, the radiation could damage the reproductive organs in either gender or the fetus in a pregnant female patient. In the brain, the radiation could change production or activity of hormones.

- If CHEMOTHERAPY is used, it could affect egg and sperm production.

This can be a time of major frustration, anger, blame, and resentment. Caregivers are impacted by these challenges as well, trying to understand the options available to them. The outcome may not be what was described to them because the treatment or the cancer may not have gone its expected course. This is doubly hard to deal with. Be sure that you have professionals to guide you through this. If you haven't talked to a specialist before treatments, there may still be time to consult one or more of these experts. The survivor's oncologist may be able to refer you to a colleague in those areas.

If you're having fertility concerns, look through some of the scenarios here. Unfortunately, there isn't space to go through every situation but you may be somewhat comforted to know that you're not alone and others have found solutions to their obstacles.

Handling Challenges With Fertility

Situation	There is a change in the desire to have or not to have children.
"We froze his sperm. The doctors told us we should do that, in case his treatment left him able to make healthy ones or have sex. It was enough to go through that. Now he's sick again, but he wants me to have them implanted and get pregnant. He wants to try to have a baby. He says he wants me to have something to remind me of him when he's gone or look forward to if he makes it. Yes, that's what he wants. Maybe I don't want to be pregnant right now. What if the pregnancy fails? Do I owe it to him to try? I don't think I'm ready. And I don't want to do it alone."	
How Can I Help?	Both people need to be in agreement when deciding to bring a child into the world and raise it. If there is an option to wait, work with your doctor, a counselor, or therapist on coming to an agreement. If not, carefully review the consequences of trying to conceive and proceed with what is right for you and the survivor.

Situation	Conception and healthy pregnancy options are limited.

"I always thought I would be a dad, a real dad, conceiving the natural way and all that. But cancer has gotten in the way. She, my wife, had ovarian and uterine cancer. All that's out now because her insides had to be taken out, you know. So they tell me to think about adoption. Now if I want a kid I have to do all this paperwork crap and get mentally evaluated and open up about my money situation and all that. I know it's not her fault, but I shouldn't be punished. She can't have a kid, but I can find somebody else who can."

How Can I Help?	There are still multiple options for having a child, including the use of egg donors (to enable conception with the partner's sperm), surrogate mothers (to carry a baby with the survivor's or donor's eggs), and adoption. Work with professionals that you trust to find the right solution for your situation.
Situation	Conception options are limited because of treatments to the male survivor and his sperm was not frozen.

"I had real concerns about going to a sperm bank. I mean, you can pick some things about the sperm to a degree, like race, but I really wanted our child to look part like David. I couldn't picture what it – our child – would look like with a sperm donor. We ended up doing it though, because you really can't choose what they look like the other way and it certainly beat the alternative of not having children at all."

How Can I Help?	Sperm donors (to enable conception with the partner's egg) and adoption are two options that you still can pursue. Again, work with professionals that you trust to find the right solution for your situation.

Situation	The physical abilities of the survivor are temporarily or permanently changed or mobility is a problem.
"We had to ask really hard questions, like: Should we even try to have a baby, knowing it could severely impact her health? Will the she be able to carry a baby to term? Who will take care of the child if she dies or is permanently confined to her bed? We decided against trying for now, because it was more important for us to have a healthy 'her' and we could always play with our friends' kids while she healed."	
How Can I Help?	It can be incredibly upsetting to watch the patient be physically altered to the point that regular routine is difficult. Sexual activity can be difficult if there are physical constraints. Pregnancy, delivery, and child rearing can be difficult as well. Physical and occupational therapists are trained to provide ways to increase strength and flexibility in survivors. Your doctors and medical staff have many options to help you according to the survivor's challenges.
Situation	Everything appears to be normal after a cancer treatment, but the couple is still not able to conceive.
"Frankly, I want to know. What the hell is the problem? Is it her or me? What can I do? "	
How Can I Help?	Stress can tremendously impact both partners physically, mentally, and emotionally. Perhaps you can find or create a relaxing environment that removes stressors for a while. Or perhaps you can work on another goal to take your mind off the fertility challenge. The timing may just not be right.

Fertility is an intense and complex issue that is best managed with medical professionals involved. Get referrals, and find people highly-trained in the specialty that you and the survivor need. Make sure that you are comfortable talking with them and that you trust them. These are serious, life-altering decisions and you want to surround yourself with the best help you can.

Juggling Work Responsibilities

"My son seems to be healed, but I still have reservations about him going back to work," says Andre, 56. "I'd just as soon as see him at home than back in the hospital if he pushes himself too hard."

Most survivors don't work during recovery from surgery, although some work through chemotherapy and radiation because of the duration of these treatments. It may be difficult to work, but concerns of employment and bill-paying do come up.

Everyone recognizes that money is important to our daily lives. Cancer survivors often feel guilty about money because the cancer consumed financial resources. When a person fights a serious illness, not only is his earning potential negatively impacted (or eliminated), but the associated costs can financially bankrupt him. Additionally, long-term impacts like lost savings, unpaid loans, and new equipment or prescription costs can be troublesome. Survivors may sense resentment at these hardships and they may feel forced to go back to work.

You may be able to help the survivor make some decisions. To help determine when he is able to go back to work (whether part-time or full-time) and if he can manage the job responsibilities consider:

- His physical state vs. the physical demands of the job

- How intense his treatment was and his doctor's recommendations

- How much flexibility he has in his job

- His emotional preparedness

- Your financial situation.

Each person's situation is different. While you want to encourage the survivor to return to work in his normal routine, you also want to be sure that the time and circumstances are right. Some survivors may feel comfortable returning to the job they've maintained for years. There they know they can find close friends, familiar surroundings, and familiar routines. In these environments, there is often some flexibility for follow-up, not to mention the continuity of insurance benefits. Plus, it's not always easy to find a new job.

However, caregivers may want to encourage survivors (and themselves!) to think about new employment. A new job means a fresh start, without constant reminders of cancer. Changing employment may be in order for many reasons:

- He is no longer able to perform the job to expected levels. He needs his responsibilities (and possibly pay) adjusted.

- He will not have to be the subject of office gossip.

- He wants more job satisfaction.

- At a new job, he will not have to disclose MEDICAL HISTORY unless additional treatment is needed or the effects will impact his job performance.

- He wants a new career, doing something he really loves.

Whether the survivor stays in his current position or moves to a new one, there will be obstacles related to his recent illness. Possible solutions are discussed in this next table.

Handling Challenges on the Job

Situation	How Can I Help?
Survivor is fully capable of returning to work but does not want to go.	If the survivor was the financial provider, gently remind him of this as well as the consequences of what happens as he waits. If possible, discuss how you can contribute financially.
Survivor wants to go back to work against doctor's orders.	Ask his supervisor to modify workload or schedule until the survivor is ready for full responsibilities. Be prepared if the survivor has a relapse or is incapable of the job requirements and cannot work until he is fully healed.
Survivor experiences employment discrimination at current job or new job.	The survivor needs to work with the human resources department or an employee representative to document and counter this in his current job. However, it's difficult to overcome and he may need to look for a new job. It's more important to try to work out the differences in a new job, as it took some effort to find this one. The survivor needs to understand the source of discrimination, especially since this is a new environment and not everyone knows the details of the illness. He needs to end the discrimination as mentioned above or move on to another job.
Survivor experiences difficulty in obtaining or retaining health or life insurance.	There's no easy answer for this. Most insurance agencies consider him a statistical high risk. Encourage him to look for work in large companies whose group insurance rarely excludes employees with a history of illness. Look for professional groups, fraternal, or political organizations that lobby to secure health insurance for previously-diagnosed survivors.

Situation	How Can I Help?
Financial compensation is decreased along with responsibilities. Disability insurance may be terminated with the return to work.	This is a huge problem, but many companies feel justified doing this. Their rationale is that they may need to hire another to handle the responsibilities that the survivor used to handle. The termination of financial support through the disability insurance can be a big blow as well. If these are happening at the same time, not returning to work may seem like the best choice. First, ask the survivor to work with his supervisor or HR on career path that will lead him back to where he was financially and professionally.

Often, the caregiver and survivor feel pressure to continue working as they did before the illness because of the flood of medical bills. Managing these bills can be a full-time job in itself. If there is interaction with the insurance companies, various medical entities, transportation groups, and labs, it can take days to answer a single question. It can be very discouraging to be approached with expenses that insurance companies won't pay and some people are overwhelmed at trying to get their arms around what they truly owe.

How Can I Help? Managing Survivor Paperwork

Here are ten things you can do when handling medical expenses:

1. Make copies of all bills and keep the originals to track what you've paid.

2. When looking at the amount of the bill, check to see if you were billed twice for the same procedure. Some offices send multiple bills for one procedure to keep you informed of their dealings with insurance.

3. Make sure all medical procedures were coded correctly. This is a common reason why insurance companies refuse to pay bills.

4. Handle bills as quickly as possible. If claims pile up, they could damage your credit.

5. Identify a contact person who is available after 5 p.m., so that you can handle things in the evening.

6. When collectors call or write, explain the situation. They may give you more time.

7. Keep trying for coverage or get an explanation of rejection. Visit a benefits administrator at work to help you understand what the insurance company is saying.

8. Ask for help from the billing department at the hospital or the doctor's office. They may refer you to other organizations that can help.

9. Some hospitals have advocacy groups to help deal with the financial impacts of the illness. Try working with a case manager or a social worker.

10. Check with your hospital to see if there are any grants or special needs programs that can help you and your family to deal with these issues.

A Few Words on Special Financial Concerns for You

No matter how much you planned or budgeted, unexpected expenses may pop up. If they don't put you in financial difficulty, they could limit your cash outlay.

It may be time to review your own employment and responsibilities. You probably need a break, but could that be in the form of new environment? A new job sometimes represents a breath of fresh air, not to mention better earning opportunities.

Use the same factors to estimate your potential for a new job: What are the physical demands of the job? How emotionally prepared are you? How much flexibility is in the schedule? Will it really improve your lifestyle or your financial situation? What are your immediate instincts about it? You may just have the ability now to pursue a dream that was previously put on hold because of this disease.

Changing Spiritual Perspectives

After treatment, both you and the patient may experience more changes in spiritual perspective. Now that it's over, you may rethink your relationship with a higher power once again. What was your relationship and where is it now? Are you fluctuating between thankfulness and anger? Does the survivor have a nothing-can-stop-me-now attitude? Are you both searching for peace?

Like other times in this caregiving journey, questions about your spirituality may surface. These are common and normal and can only be answered by the individual. Devote what time you need to address them.

Celebrating with the Survivor

With successful outcomes, most people have a degree of thankfulness that can be shared. If there are others around, ask them for assistance in planning a little event. You've been through a big experience and even though there may still be some challenges, you should enjoy the good that's happened. Try these suggestions:

- Enjoy the sunshine! Keep the survivor's room well lit and ventilated. Go for a walk together.

- Stage a little homecoming with streamers and balloons or a special meal.

- Sing with the survivor. Children's songs like "The Itsy Bitsy Spider" or "I'm a Little Teapot" can be comforting and fun. Or, if you're looking for celebration tunes, how about "I Feel Good," "Looks Like We Made It" or "We Are The Champions."

- Bring back more touching into your routine. Encourage hugging, hand-holding, or snuggling as appropriate.

- As the survivor heals, try to dance, first with gentle steps and then more vigorous ones as with the Hokey Pokey.

You may have your own private ways to celebrate, and that's terrific. Do whatever makes you feel good about your accomplishment and your lives. That's between you and the survivor.

Taking Care of Yourself

"One day, the doctor called me. He told me John was NED. No Evidence of Disease," says Kerry, 55. "I was freed! No more care giving. But then, like the prisoner who goes out into the real world, I was stunned. I didn't know how to act anymore or what to do. In a weird way, I longed for the comfort of my jail confinement. He's elated and going on with his new life. All I can think about is the way it was. And what do I do now?"

It's time for you to take a breather.

As the survivor finishes treatment and has gotten a good report from the doctor, it's time to take a look at all that you have done. You have done a wonderful job of filling all the roles that come along with being a caregiver. It's time to begin your transition back to life without those roles.

Creating a New Role for You, the Caregiving Survivor

After you experience the stamp of cancer on your life, it's difficult to 'remove the ink,' so to speak. It seems to leave a lasting mark no matter how you try to remove it. More often than not, it seems that little good can come from a cancer experience. Yet it's difficult to move on.

You may not be able to let go of the worry. Guilt and regrets may arise. Undoubtedly, you will have felt some anger along the caregiving path. You're also likely to be coping with fear of the disease spreading or coming back. Those fears and insecurities may be stressful to hide, but they are also stressful to discuss. You may want to leave all this behind but you find it impossible.

It's very common to feel caught between two worlds. Ironically, when the survivor seems to have fewer problems, you may be struggling with conflicting thoughts and feelings. You must release the old roles and find a new pattern of daily life in relation to his. You've got to encourage the survivor to be as strong as he can be on his own. Sooner than later, you've got to get out of the caregiver role and into your survivor mode.

You need to assess what's right for you, as far as how you transition away from caregiving and into your own routine. When you decide that you're ready to proceed, go for it. Leave the guilt and the worry behind. The next sections will give you some direction on how to make your new life happen.

As you're creating the new role for yourself, keep this new title in mind: Caregiving Survivor. You will continue to give care, to yourself and to others when you can. You are a survivor, not from the illness, but from the many impacts that this illness has had on you. You've weathered this storm and you'll handle another one like a pro if it comes up. This kind of thing won't get you down. You are a Caregiving Survivor.

What does that mean? It simply means that what you chose to do from here on in will fall into one or both of those categories. You'll make the choices that are right for your life. You'll think of options and surround yourself with a support team if adversity shows itself again.

How will you do this? By now, you're familiar with the advice from other Caregiving Survivors. They have shared their wisdom with you from the beginning of this book, and want to give a little more at the end. They suggest that you:

- Accept and rejoice in your life as it is now. Choose things you enjoy and don't be afraid to try new things.

- Give yourself some time to heal. Appreciate yourself and what you are capable of.

- Take some recognition for your efforts, either privately or publicly. You did a lot of work. No one else did it and you deserve the credit.

- Spend time with people who are supportive. Some people will not understand the toll this experience has taken on you. Try to ignore them.

Lastly, don't give up. You may choose to give care to another person or even the same person going through more treatments or multiple cancers. Keep your head up and know that you're strong. You've survived this once and you really can do it again if you need to. We'll talk about goals for healthy living next.

Defining Goals for Healthy Living

As strange as this may sound, cancer can be a powerful teacher. After a diagnosis, it teaches many life lessons. Cancer teaches us about our vulnerabilities and our strengths. It helps us identify who and what we want in our lives. Cancer introduces us to new places, people, and ideas. It propels us to try new things. Essentially, cancer forces a change in priority as we temporarily place it at the center of our lives.

Through the progression of the illness and following its treatment, cancer can also teach how to live. We are faced with questions that push us to define our reason for being. Cancer can teach us to evaluate how we fill our lives and encourages us to take responsibility for achieving our goals. If you have learned these lessons without having the disease yourself, you've increased your chances for maintaining healthy living.

Now we can reprioritize our lives, no longer placing cancer at the center. We must allow ourselves to let go of the trauma and to move forward. Many people consider this a second chance at life. But how do you go about deciding what you're going to do with this second chance?

Sometimes things just fall into place. Other times, you may need to be proactive. If being proactive is for you, start by thinking about what you want. Ask yourself how you see your future. If you have an idea of your new purpose and can clearly see your goals, break them down into steps and put them in action. If you don't have an idea of your new purpose, take your time and think about it. Consider what you'd like your relationships, your daily living, your employment situation, and your spirituality to be. Salvage what you want from the past and don't be afraid to start fresh. Use any resources you can to define your goals for healthy living.

When you figure out your goals, start slowly and with someone who genuinely wants you to succeed. In the best circumstances, caregivers and survivors have goals that are aligned, in terms of focus and timeline. Write them down and work on them together. If your goals are not aligned, work with a partner or a friend who offers support, accountability, and sometimes a little competition.

In your new life, remember the "healthy" part of healthy living. Neither you nor the survivor should act in an extreme manner because of newly-found freedom, energy, or acceptance of mortality. Use that motivation to achieve what you want to achieve, but be aware of the power and the limitations of your own efforts. Try beginning small, at home, with the goals in your daily routine. Then, build on those successes and take your motivation out into the world.

Wrapping Up

You've done a great job at managing all the changes that come with cancer treatment. In many ways, living with outcomes after treatment is similar to living with outcomes during treatment. In this chapter, we looked at solutions for obstacles that follow treatment such as eating, moving, and sharing affection. We talked about the transition from being a patient to being a survivor.

You're beginning to understand where you fit into the patient's post-treatment life. You're ready to transition from those old roles and into a new one. In reviewing your roles and responsibilities, you've taken on a lot. As your caregiving journey comes to a close, you've got the tools to move from the role of caregiver to caregiving survivor.

Welcome to the final destination on your caregiving journey.

You've defined some goals for healthy living and with this incredible experience under your belt, the world is your oyster. Hold your head high and go after what you want to accomplish. You can do it.

Resource Directory

Many resources exist to help you on your caregiving journey. You may find assistance through local organizations, such as public libraries (which also provide internet access), houses of worship, the local newspaper, or service and senior groups. Several regional and national organizations are contained in these pages to give you additional options for assistance.

Please note: While every attempt has been made to ensure the accuracy of contact information, changes happen over time. We provide this directory as a service to you and have no connection to the operation of these organizations. The directory is not intended as an endorsement or recommendation for any treatment, product, service, or activity.

General Cancer Information, Support Groups, and Free Services

- American Cancer Society, www.cancer.org, 800-ACS-2345 (or 800-227-2345)

- Cancer*Care,* www.cancercare.org, 800-813-HOPE (or 800-813-4673)

- Cancer Information Service at The National Cancer Institute, www.cancer.gov, 800-4-CANCER (or 800-422-6237)

- Lance Armstrong Foundation, www.livestrong.org, 866-235-7205

- National Center for Complementary and Alternative Medicine (NCCAM) at the National Institutes of Health, www.nih.gov/about/almanac/organization/NCCAM.htm, 888-644-6226 or 301-496-4000

- National Coalition for Cancer Survivorship (NCCS), www.canceradvocacy.org, 301-650-9127

- National Health Information Center, www.health.gov/nhic/, 800-336-4797

- Post-Treatment Resource Program, Memorial Sloan-Kettering Cancer Center, www.mskcc.org, 212-717-3527

Specific Illness Information

Bladder Cancer

- Bladder Cancer Advocacy Network, www.bcan.org, 301-469-6865

- M.D. Anderson Bladder Cancer Support Team, www.mdanderson.org/departments/bladdercansup/, 800-392-1611

Breast Cancer

- Men Against Breast Cancer, www.menagainstbreastcancer.org, 866-547-MABC (or 866-547-6222)

- National Alliance of Breast Cancer Organizations Through NCCS, www.NABCO.org, 301-650-9127

- Susan G. Komen for the Cure, cms.komen.org, 800 I'M AWARE (or 800-462-9273)

Colon/Rectal Cancer

- Colorectal Cancer Alliance, www.ccalliance.org, 301-879-1500

- Colorectal Cancer Network, www.colorectalcancer.net, 877-422-2030

Lung Cancer

- Alliance for Lung Cancer Advocacy, Support, and Education, www.lungcanceralliance.org, 202-463-2080

- It's Time to Focus on Lung Cancer, www.lungcancer.org, 877-646-LUNG (or 877-646-5864)

Pancreatic Cancer

- Pancreatica, www.pancreatica.com, 831-658-0600

- Pancreatic Cancer Action Network www.PanCAN.org, 877-272-9227

- Patient and Liaison Services (PALS), 877-272-6226

Prostate Cancer

- Man to Man, American Cancer Society, www.cancer.acs, 800-ACS-2345 (or 800-227-2345)

- Prostate Pointers/Us Too!, www.prostatepointers.org, (No phone number at this time)

Skin Cancers

- American Melanoma Foundation, www.melanomafoundation.org, 619-448-0991

- Skin Cancer Foundation, www.skincancer.org, 800-490-SKIN (or 800-490-7546)

Women's Reproductive Cancers

- Ovarian Cancer National Alliance, www.ovariancancer.org, 202-331-1332

- Women's Cancer Network, www.wcn.org, 312-578-1439

Fertility Concerns

- American Society for Reproductive Medicine, www.asrm.org, 205-978-5000

- FertileHOPE, www.fertilehope.org, 888-994-HOPE (or 888-994-4663)

Insurance and Benefits

A state-by-state analysis of insurance possibilities and coverage is provided by most state governments by the Insurance Commissioner. You and the patient may want to investigate options for Comprehensive Health Insurance for High Risk Individuals.

- ADA Information Line, www.ada.gov, 800-514-0301

- Consumer's Guide to Health Insurance, www.healthinsuranceinfo.net, (No phone number at this time)

- Centers for Medicare and Medicaid Services, www.cms.hhs.gov, 877-267-2323

- Department of Veterans Affairs, www.va.gov, 800-827-1000

- FMLA, www.dol.gov/esa/whd/fmla.htm, 866-4US-WAGE (or 866-487-9243)

- Medicare Information, www.medicare.gov, 800-MEDICARE (or 800-633-4227)

- EAP (Employee Assistance Programs), www.eap.sap.com, Phone numbers are available for specific programs through the employer.

- Social Security Administration, www.ssa.gov, 800-772-1213

Drug Companies with Patient Assistance Programs

- Bristol Myers Squibb, www.TogetherRxAccess.com, 800-444-4106

- Eli Lilly Patient Assistance, Lillly Cares Program, www.lillycares.com, 800-545-6962

- Partnership for Prescription Assistance, www.pparx.org, 888-477-2669

- Wyeth Pharmaceuticals Patient Assistance Program, www.wyeth.com, 800-568-9938

Mental Health, Pain Management, and Stress Management Resources

- American Academy of Pain Management, www.aapainmanage.org/, 209-533-9744

- The Center for Loss and Bereavement, www.bereavementcenter.org, 610-222-4110

- International Stress Management Association (ISMA) www.apa.org/journals/str, 800-374-2721

- National Suicide Prevention Lifeline, www.suicidepreventionlifeline.org, 800-273-TALK (or 800-273-8255)

- National Institute of Mental Health, National Institutes of Health, www.nimh.nih.gov/, 866-615-6464

- Shanti Project, www.shanti.org, 415-674-4700

Respite Care

Each state government has an Office on Aging that may have suggestions on respite care for caregivers. You may want to contact your state or local government directory listings for more information.

- AmeriCare Alliance, www.americarealliance.com, 800-610-2029

- Visiting Angels, www.visitingangels.com, 800-365-4189

Retreats and Activities

- A New Beginning Cancer Retreat, www.cancer-retreat.org, 641-772-4276

- Camp Make-A-Dream (children), www.campdream.org, 406-549-5987

- Camp Sunshine (children), www.mycampsunshine.com, 404-325-7979

- Commonweal Cancer Help Program, www.commonweal.org, 415-868-0970

- First Descents (teenagers), www.firstdescents.org, 970-328-1806

- Life Beyond Cancer, www.lifebeyondcancer.com, lifebeyondcancer@usoncology.com, (No phone number at this time)

- Ski to Live, www.kristenulmer.com, 801-733-5003

- Smith Farm Cancer Help Program, www.smithfarm.com, 202-483-8600

- Sunstone Cancer Support Foundation, www.sunstonehealing.net, 520-749-1928

- The Wellness Community, www.wellnesscommunity.org, 888-793-WELL (or 888-793-9355)

Additional Web Sites

The Compassionate Caregiver's web site is an online resource for caregivers at www.compassionatecaregiveronline.com. Other resources you may be interested in are listed below.

- Air Transportation for the Cancer Patient or Family: www.corpangelnetwork.org

- Cancer Net: www.cancer.gov/cancer information

- Cancer Research Institute: www.cancerresearch.org

- Caregiver Discounts, Resources: www. caregiversmarketplace.com

- Caregiver Support: www.caringinfo.org

- Caregiver Support: www.strengthforcaring.com

- Caregiving Tips: www.caregiver.com

- Family Caregiver Alliance: www.caregiver.org

- Home Health Care Providers: www.home-health-care.biz

- Indigent Medication Resources: www.indicare.com

- Indigent Medication Resources: www.needymeds.com

- Indigent Medication Resources: www.themedicineprogram.com

- National Alliance for Caregiving: www.caregiving.org

- National Family Caregiver's Association: www.nfcacares.org

- Pain Management: www.stoppain.org

- Research News: www.cancernews.com

- Wishes for Future Care: www.findingourway.net

- Wishes for Future Care: www.lastacts.org

- Wishes for Future Care: www.agingwithdignity.org/5wishes.html

Recommended Reading

- Bombeck, Erma. <u>Forever, Erma: Best-Loved Writing from America's Favorite Humorist</u>. Kansas City, MO: Andrew McMeel Universal Company,1996.

- DeKlyen, Chuck and Pat Schwiebert. <u>Tear Soup</u>. Portland, OR: Griefwatch, 2001.

- Hutchison, Joyce and Rupp, Joyce. <u>May I Walk You Home? Courage and Comfort for Caregivers of the Very Ill</u>. Notre Dame, IN: Ave Maria Press, 1999.

- Hyde, Susan Sturges. <u>No More Bad-Hair Days</u>. Atlanta, GA: Longstreet Press, 1996.

- Remen, Rachel Naomi. <u>Kitchen Table Wisdom</u>. New York, NY: Riverhead Books, 1996.

Other Components of The Compassionate Caregiver Series®

If you've found this guide helpful, you might be interested in other tools and support from The Compassionate Caregiver Series®. Visit the web site for more resources, including upcoming handbooks in these areas:

- Understanding the Cancer Diagnosis

- Palliative and Hospice Care

- When Cancer Claims the Life

- The Journey of Grief.

Find us on the internet at www.CompassionateCaregiverOnline. com. Email your suggestions for the next edition of this book to bonnie@CompassionateCaregiverOnline.com.

Bibliography

Books

- Adrouny, A. Richard. <u>Understanding Colon Cancer</u>. Jackson, MI: University Press of Mississippi, 2002.

- The Alpha Institute. <u>The Alpha Book on Cancer and Living for Patients, Family and Friends</u>. Alameda, CA: The Alpha Institute, 1993.

- Auerbach, Michael. <u>Conversations about Cancer: A Patient's Guide to Informed Decision-Making</u>. Baltimore, MD: Williams & Wilkins, 1997.

- Babcock, Elise NeeDell. <u>When Life Becomes Precious: A Guide for Loved Ones and Friends of Cancer Patients</u>. New York, NY: Bantam Books, 1997.

- Benjamin, Harold H., Ph.D. <u>The Wellness Community: Guide to Fight for Recovery From Cancer</u>. New York, NY: Jeremy P. Archer, 1987.

- Benowitz, Steven I. <u>Cancer</u>. Springfield, NJ: Enslow Publishers, 1999.

- Bloomfield, Harold H. and Kory, Robert B. <u>The Holistic Way to Health and Happiness: A New Approach to Complete Lifetime Wellness</u>. New York, NY: Simon and Schuster, 1978.

- Buckman, Robert. <u>What You Really Need to Know About CANCER: A Comprehensive Guide for Patients and Their Families</u>. Baltimore, MD: The Johns Hopkins University Press, 1995.

- Carroll, David. Living With Dying: A Loving Guide for Family and Close Friends. New York, NY: McGraw-Hill Book Company, 1985.

- Cefrey, Holly. Coping with Cancer. New York, NY: The Rosen Publishing Group, Inc., 2000.

- Cohen, Deborah A. Just Get Me Through This! The Practical Guide to Breast Cancer. New York, NY: Kensington Publishing Corp., 2000.

- Coleman, C. Norman. Understanding Cancer: A Patient's Guide to Diagnosis, Prognosis and Treatment. Baltimore, MD: The Johns Hopkins University Press, 1998.

- Dooley, Joseph F. and Marian Betancourt. The Coming Cancer Breakthroughs. New York, NY: Kensington Publishing Corp., 2002.

- Drum, David. Making the ChemoTherapy Decision. Los Angeles, CA: Lowell House/RGA Publishing Group, 1996.

- Dunne, Jemima, Managing Editor. Visiting Nurse Associations of America Caregiver's Handbook: A Complete Guide to Home Health Care. New York: DK Publishing, Inc., 1998.

- Evans, Mark ed. Yoga, Tai Chi, Massage, Therapies & Healing Remedies -- Natural ways to health, relaxation and vitality: a complete practical guide. New York, NY: Hermes House, Anness Publishing Inc., 2002.

- Harpham, Wendy Schlessel. After Cancer: A Guide to Your New Life. New York, NY: W.W. Norton & Co., Inc., 1994.

- Harwell, Amy with Kristine Tomasik. When Your Friend Gets Cancer: How You Can Help. Wheaton, IL: Harold Shaw Publishers, 1987.

- Holland, Jimmie C. with Sheldon Lewis. <u>The Human Side of Cancer: Living with Hope, Coping with Uncertainty</u>. New York, NY: HarperCollins Publishers, Inc., 2001.

- King, Dean, et al. <u>Cancer Combat: Cancer Survivors Share Their Guerilla Tactics to Help You Win the Fight of Your Life</u>. New York, NY: Bantam Books, 1998.

- Lynn, Joanne. <u>Handbook for Mortals: Guidance for People Facing Serious Illness</u>. New York, NY: Oxford University Press, 1999.

- Natelson, Benjamin. <u>Facing and Fighting Fatigue</u>. Binghampton, NY: Vail-Ballou Press, 1998.

- Svec, Carol. <u>After Any Diagnosis</u>. New York, NY: Three Rivers Press, 2001.

- Thomas, Richard and Peter Albright, M.D. <u>The Complete Book of Natural Pain Relief: Safe and effective self-help for everyday aches and pains</u>. Buffalo, NY: Firefly Books, Inc., 1998.

- Spark, Richard F., M.D. <u>Sexual Health For Men: The Complete Guide</u>. Cambridge, MA: Perseus Publishing, 2000.

- Tannock, Ian F., et al. <u>The Basic Science of Oncology</u>. New York, NY: McGraw-Hill Medical Publishing Division, 2005.

Other Publications

- CAM at the NIH. Focus on Complementary and Alternative Medicine. Bethesda, MD. Spring 2005.

- Cleveland Clinic Magazine. Cleveland Clinic Foundation. Fertility Preservation For Cancer Patients. Cleveland, OH. Winter 2004.

- Understanding Lymphedema. Cleveland Clinic Foundation. Cleveland, OH. 1998.

- Department of Health and Human Services. Notice of Privacy Practices. Health Insurance Portability and Accountability Act. Washington, DC. April 2003.

- Hospice Foundation of America. Living with Grief: At School. A Practical Guide for Schools. Doka, Kenneth J. Washington, DC. 1999.

- Hospice Foundation of America. Living with Grief: At Work. A Practical Guide for the Workplace. Doka, Kenneth J. Washington, DC. 1999.

- Hospice Foundation of America. Living with Grief: At Worship. A Practical Guide for Faith Communities. Doka, Kenneth J. Washington, DC. 1999.

- National Coalition for Cancer Survivorship. What Cancer Survivors Need To Know About Health Insurance. Silver Springs, MD. 2003.

- National Coalition for Cancer Survivorship. Teamwork: The Cancer Patient's Guide to Talking With Your Doctor. Silver Spring, MD. 1992.

- National Institutes of Health/National Cancer Institute. What Are Clinical Trials All About? Bethesda, MD. 1997.

- National Partnership for Women and Families. Guide to the Family and Medical Leave Act. Questions and Answers. Fifth Edition. Washington, DC. 2002.

- NCBI at the National Institutes of Health. PUBMED. www.ncbi.nlm.nih.gov. Palliative care in undergraduate medical education. Status report and future directions. J.A. Billings and S. Block. Washington, DC. 1997.

- OncoLink. Web site of the University of Pennsylvania Cancer Center. www.oncolink.com. Cancer Survivorship. Linda A. Jacobs, PhD, CRNP, AOCN. Philadelphia, PA. Posted March 25, 2001. Last revision of site: Sunday, July 22, 2001.

- Pancreatic Cancer Action Network. PanCAN News. Volume III, Issue 2. El Segundo, CA: April 2003.

- The Shepherd Center. Clontz, Kim Lathbury. Hiring Help. Spinal Column. Atlanta, GA. Summer 2005.

- U.S. Department of Health and Human Services. Managing Cancer Pain. Washington, DC. Public Health Service. 1994.

- U.S. Equal Employment Opportunity Commission. U.S. Department of Justice Civil Rights Division. Washington, DC. Americans with Disabilities Act Questions and Answers from www.usdoj.gov/crt/ada. 2005.

- U.S. Social Security Administration Medicare and Medicaid. Medicare and You. Washington, DC. 2005.

- The Wellness Community. Open to Options. Cancer Clinical Trials. Washington, DC. 2003.

Presentations

- "Breakthroughs in Radiology" by 20th Century Radiology. As presented at the 17th Annual Western North Carolina Cancer Conference, Asheville, NC 2005.

- "Cancer Survival Toolbox: Basic Skills" cassettes distributed by National Coalition for Cancer Survivorship. Washington, DC 1998.

- "Compassion Fatigue," by Karl D. La Rowe, MA, LCSW. As presented through PESI HealthCare in Atlanta, GA 2005.

- "Managing Difficult Patient Situations," by Rachel Boersma. As presented through PESI HealthCare in Atlanta, GA 2005.

- "Strength 4 Your Journey: Taking Control of Cancer" CD-ROM distributed by Ortho BioTech. Bridgewater, NJ 2004.

Glossary

This glossary includes terms associated with cancer that appear throughout this book.

In the interest of simplicity, each is given a brief description, which has been provided by members of the Medical Advisory Board. For more information, go to www.cancer.gov for the National Cancer Institute Dictionary of Cancer Terms.

Adjuvant Therapy – Treatment or therapy given to a patient after a primary therapy to decrease the potential of recurrence. Usually, it is given after the cancer has been completely removed by surgery.

Advance Directive Documents (also called Advance Directives) – Formal documents containing the patient's wishes for future healthcare.

Alopecia – Loss of hair. When used in reference to cancer, it is usually associated with hair loss that may appear as a side effect of chemotherapy. In this case, the hair usually grows back.

Anemia – When the level of red blood cells in the blood is below normal. This can cause fatigue in the patient.

Aromatase Inhibitor – A type of chemotherapy given by mouth to treat breast cancer.

Aspiration – When contents from the stomach go into the lungs and cause coughing.

Biopsy – When tissues are removed for diagnosis.

Blood Counts (also called CBC) – A laboratory measurement of the blood cells obtained from a blood specimen. These cells are the erythrocytes (red blood cells or RBC), leukocytes (white blood cells or WBC) and platelets.

Cancer Cells (also called Malignant Cells or Tumors) – Cells in the body that are abnormal in size, color, texture, or function whose unrestricted growth patterns are harmful to other systems or organs.

Care Plan – The medical and non-medical steps that caregivers take, the services caregivers use, and the organizations that caregivers involve to care for the cancer patient.

Care Team – Medical and non-medical people who support caregivers in getting the patient good care.

Chemotherapy – A type of treatment with drugs (also called chemicals or agents), that can be administered by mouth, intravenously, or injection into the tissues.

Chemo Brain – A recognized effect of chemotherapy on the patient where cognitive (or thinking) abilities are temporarily impaired.

Clinical Trials – Research studies that evaluate the safety and effectiveness of potential new treatments or medicines.

Compassion Fatigue – Lack of energy brought on by insufficient sleep, emotional distress, and lack of nutrition.

CT Scan (also pronounced CAT Scan) – Short for Computerized Axial Tomography. Multiple X-rays obtained from a 360° circle around the patient are assembled by the computer into a series of three dimensional "slices" of the body.

Cycle – One complete course of chemotherapy.

Debulking – Surgical removal or destruction of the majority of, but not all of, a tumor.

Deep Vein Thrombosis – A blood clot inside a vessel.

Diagnosis – A tentative or definitive determination of cause(s) of a medical problem made from information provided by patient history, physical exam, laboratory or imaging (X-Ray, CT, or MRI) studies. It states what the doctors are expecting before tissues are tested and the reports come back from the pathologists.

DNR (Short for <u>D</u>o <u>N</u>ot <u>R</u>esuscitate) – An Advance Directive document that outlines the patient's wishes to limit the start or scope of life-support treatment.

External Beam – A type of radiation from a machine outside the patient's body.

Field of Radiation – The area or part of the body treated by radiation therapy.

First Line Therapy – The initial chemotherapy regimen used for treatment, usually with the most effective current drug or combination of drugs.

Graft vs. Host Disease – An attempt by the new bone marrow (graft) to reject the patient's normal tissues (host) following a bone marrow transplant.

HIPAA (Health Insurance Portability and Accountability Act) – The national act to protect patient privacy of health-related information and to enable insurance coverage to continue through a job change or job loss.

Hospice – A program of comfort care and support services for patients with a life-limiting progressive illness who are no longer seeking curative care. It supports their families and loved ones as well.

Immunotherapy – A type (or modality) of treatment that involves biological substances. These substances have a direct tumor-killing effect or enhance the killing effects of the normal immune system. Immunotherapy can be administered by mouth, intravenously or injection into the tissues.

Implant – A type of radiation where the source is inserted into the patient's body.

Incision Site – Site of the opening in the tissues, usually in the skin, through which surgery is performed.

Intravenous (IV) – When a liquid form of medication, food, or treatment is delivered directly into a patient's bloodstream (circulation) through a vein.

Intubation – In general, placing a tube into a body structure. It usually refers to placing of a tube in the trachea ("wind pipe") to breathe for a patient.

Late Effects – Changes in the patient happening as a direct result of treatment which may appear years after the treatment has finished. After effects happen commonly with radiation. For example, a patient receiving radiation may experience poor wound healing years later. See also Side Effects.

Localized – Treatment directed only at the site of the tumor. This is in contrast to treatment like chemotherapy when given to entire body ("systemic therapy").

Lymphatic System – A system of lymph nodes, channels and organs including the spleen, liver and bone marrow.

Lymphedema – Swelling of an extremity like the arms or legs.

Margin – The rim of tissue around a tumor that is surgically removed along with the tumor during surgery. This margin is tested by pathologists to assist in determining if all the cancer cells have been removed.

Mastectomy – A surgical treatment for breast cancer removing the entire breast.

Medical History – The patient's medical background. It includes a general review of the current problem and symptoms of the patient; details of any previous surgeries, procedures or diseases; family history and social history; and current medications and allergies.

Metastasis – The ability of the cancer to spread "discontinuously" beyond the original tumor site, through the blood, the lymphatic system or a body cavity.

Minimally-Invasive – A type of surgery using smaller incisions performed inside a body cavity using a video camera and instruments passed into the cavity through tubes called "ports."

Modality – A type of treatment such as surgery, radiation, or chemotherapy.

MRI – Short for Magnetic Resonance Imaging. X-ray test where signals from the body's molecules are collected after exposure to a strong magnetic field. Signals are fed into a computer that interprets them and presents the results as a 3-D slice of the body.

Multimodal Therapy (also called Multimodality) – Any or all of major forms of treatment or therapy may be used together or in sequence to treat a patient's disease.

Neoadjuvant Therapy – A type (or modality) of treatment given in preparation for the primary treatment or therapy. An example would be radiation before surgery to shrink the tumor size.

Neuropathy – Injury to the patient's nervous system usually apparent in the hands or feet, such as tingling, numbness, pain, or "pins and needles."

Node – A part of the lymphatic system that may be removed to detect the spread of cancer.

Oncology – The study of cancer.

Open Surgery – Abdominal or chest surgery performed through a large incision with the surgeon working within the body cavity.

Ostomy – A surgically created opening of the intestine onto the abdominal wall to remove urine or feces from the body.

Palliative Care – A program of care to relieve suffering and manage symptoms but not necessary to cure the disease.

Pathology Report – A formal report issued after tissue samples are analyzed by physicians.

Portacath – A completely intravenous device implanted in the patient, usually in the chest, which enables medical professionals to draw blood and to give medicine without individual needle sticks. This may be used in chemotherapy.

PRN (Short for <u>P</u>ro <u>Re</u> <u>Na</u>ta) – Often contained in doctor's orders or on prescriptions, this is an abbreviation meaning "as needed."

Prognosis – The likely chance for recovery or recurrence if the disease follows its normal course. These can be given with and without consideration of treatment impacts.

Protocol – Detailed plans of treatment including procedures, tests and follow-up, sometimes referred to as Regimen.

Radiation Therapy (also called Radiotherapy or Radiation) – A type (or modality) of treatment using high-energy rays (x-rays or gamma rays) for cancer treatment. Radiation can be used as the main treatment, to reduce the size of a tumor before surgery, or to reduce some of the symptoms of cancer. It can be given externally or implanted internally.

Radioprotector – Substance applied to the skin to prevent injury from radiation therapy.

Reconstruction – Surgical rebuilding of the tissues lost after radiation or another surgery.

Recurrence (also called Relapse) – Return of cancer or signs of cancer.

Regimen – The specific dose, schedule and duration of treatment, often used to describe a chemotherapy approach.

Relapse – See Recurrence.

Remission – The period of time when the cancer is responding to treatment or is under control.

Resectible – A pre-operative assessment that the tumor is completely removable by surgery.

Resection – Surgical removal of tissue.

Side Effects – Problems caused by cancer treatments affecting healthy cells at the same time or shortly after treatments or prescriptions. See also Late Effects.

Simulation – Detailed planning of radiation treatment from CT scan images, using sophisticated computerized programs.

Standard of Care – Accepted methods of care to treat an illness or injury that cause the least harm and bring the greatest benefit to the patient.

Surgery – Manual procedure(s) to sample, remove, or treat the effects of cancers on the body.

Survival Rates – A statistical benchmark chosen to evaluate overall survival from a clinical point, such as the beginning of treatment. Survival rates are the percentage of people who have survived a given cancer up to a given time. These rates are measured in periods covering 1, 2, 3, 5, and 10 years from the start of treatment.

Systemic – Treatment given to entire body. It is the opposite of localized treatment.

Tissue – Part of the body that will be removed in a biopsy or other surgery to provide information on the tumor.

Toxicity – Adverse effects of a treatment. These are usually temporary.

Tumor – An abnormal mass of tissue.

Tumor-Node-Metastasis (TNM) – A description of the cancer used to determine the prognosis and treatment.

Index

284

Printed in the United States
74410LV00005B/97-240

9 781425 989743